BOSS *to*
BIKINI

BOSS *to* BIKINI

The Bikini Boss Complete Transformation Program

THERESA
DEPASQUALE

A POST HILL PRESS BOOK
ISBN: 978-1-61868-817-0
ISBN (eBook): 978-1-61868-816-3

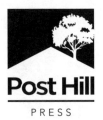

Post Hill Press
275 Madison Avenue, 14th Floor
New York, NY 10016
http://posthillpress.com

Dedication

This book is dedicated to the women who truly want to improve their lives and bodies for the better; for those who are seeking to learn and take control of their health. It's not easy, but it's definitely worth it. I have massive respect for you and your determination. I wrote this book to give you the tools and resources that have helped me radically change my body and life and I hope it will help you do the same.

Author's Note

Those of you who already know me know that I tell it like it is. When I feel strongly about something, I'm very direct and use profanity. If you're offended easily, this may not be the book for you. But I would say the same things if we were having a conversation.

Acknowledgments

I would like to give special thanks to my husband, Vincent, for supporting me as I went through this process and allowing me to follow my passion. I love you.

I owe a huge thank you to Dr. Moses Bernard who has helped me with the research and development for all Bikini Boss Fitness LLC programs and services, including the 90-day transformation program included in this book. He has had an immense influence on me throughout the past decade and I greatly admire his commitment to training and education. I feel lucky and honored to call you a close friend and colleague. THANK YOU.

Contents

Boss to Bikini
90-DAY WORKOUT PROGRAM

BOSS *to* BIKINI

#Big Girl Pants On

PART

1

Becoming Your Own Boss

CONGRATULATIONS! YOU'RE BUSY. I get it. So are the rest of the 126,675,923 women who go to work every single day and deal with the same shit. If you want to become a Bikini Boss—and I mean really WANT to become a Bikini Boss—there is one position you need to own like you're getting paid Bill Gates-style to own it, and that's your life!

BYOB. Although I know the college sorority girl inside of you just reminisced for a second, we are not talking about alcoholic beverages here; we are talking about your life. We are talking about your goals and aspirations. If you want to get to the next level—if you want to stop talking the same crap over and over and instead start getting results—it all starts with *BYOB, Becoming Your Own Boss*. Stop and really think about this statement for a second. Ask yourself how you're able to manage your house, your kids, your pets, your career, your employees, your social life—but you can't seem to get your own act together enough to stick to any kind of a schedule or make time for yourself? You and I both know the answer to this question. It's because you have not fully accepted this position. You have not yet committed to owning the most important position you will ever have and that's being the CEO of your life. YOU are the person in charge of yourself and until you accept this fact, your life will continue to run you.

INITIATIVE— (/iˈniSH(ē)ədv/) the power or opportunity to act or take charge before others do.

I would like to first redefine this word to a meaning I feel is more apt for this discussion—which is "the first step to putting your big girl pants on." In order to be a Bikini Boss you need to put on your big girl pants and start doing things for yourself. While we're growing up we have mommy, daddy and grandma to constantly guide us and tell us what we should or should not be doing, when to do it, and even sometimes where. Then suddenly at some point in our lives they throw us to the proverbial wolves and we are left to adjust to this newfound freedom either by stepping up to the challenge or falling apart! In most cases, unfortunately, I think it's the latter.

Luckily for me, my parents taught me to be pretty self-sufficient at a young age, so I learned that if I wanted things done I had to do them myself. This included things like buying nice clothes, going places, and even buying my first car. As much as I resented it back then, simply for the fact all the other parents bought their kids the cool clothes and nice cars for their birthdays, I could not be more thankful for it now. These lessons taught me if I wanted something it was up to ME to get it. It taught me personal responsibility. And that is hands down one of the most important lessons of my life.

Take note: If you're one of those people who grew up on the other end of the spectrum and had everything pretty much given to you, don't worry! I won't lie—it's going to take a lot more work and mental fortitude for you to adopt these new belief systems and habits into your life, but once you do, it's pretty much game over! You will feel more accomplished and find more fulfillment than you ever have before and the satisfaction of being in charge of yourself will be completely empowering and addicting.

FIRST THINGS FIRST

In order to accomplish anything in life, you need to set goals. I'm sure you often have heard this before, especially if you've reached any level of success, but the reality is goal setting works and you need to do it. Period. I assume many readers are already familiar with this concept—at least with regard to your career—but if for some reason you're not translating this practice to your life, we need to change this.

I am not going to tell you to follow a specific exercise for goal setting because I think different individuals respond better to different methods; however, I will tell you there is a definite benefit to taking the time to clearly outline and visualize exactly what you want AND how you will get it.

My experience with goal setting has been atypical since I do not partake in the daily exercises recommended by most experts. To be totally honest, I can barely make it out of the house on time with the kids every morning, let alone have the time to do a whole goal-setting ritual! I can tell you this though; regardless of how often I revisit my goals, once I write them down and visualize them—they do happen eventually. Even though I do not look at my goal book every day, the mere act of writing and visualizing it as if it was already happening sends a signal to the universe and more importantly plants a seed in my brain which somehow always helps to make sure my actions are aligned with my goals. If you ask anyone who has reached even the most basic level of success, he or she will tell you the same thing— goal setting works.

A few things to keep in mind when you're writing out your goals: EVERYTHING TAKES TIME, and usually way more time than you initially planned or expected it to take. It doesn't matter if it's your personal goals, fitness or business goals, it is not going to be an overnight process. Be realistic or you will set yourself up for failure from the start. And keep this in mind: I guarantee, even if you don't hit your goals in the timeframe you have listed, you will have made great progress and will be much closer to hitting them had you done nothing or never spelled out your goals in the first place.

As I mentioned, there are many ways to do goal-setting exercises but I'll briefly touch on the two which have worked well for me and hopefully these will spark some ideas and/or create enough initiative for you to do your own goal setting.

VISION BOARDS

I'm talking cool vision boards—ones with stuff on it that actually mean something to you and have some kind of emotional connection, not just scraps you pasted on from a cheesy activity you did at your last work pow wow. I'm sure some of you have made a vision board in the past and if you're like me, you threw it in the back of the closet and never looked at it at it again. That's because you didn't take it seriously or take the time to make one that meant anything to you. First, make a board that has some meaningful stuff on it! Take time and collect images that are things you really want out of life. Look for pictures or objects you can relate to and picture for yourself, not some silly arbitrary images that for some may imply success. Secondly, put it where you can see it. Mine is in my closet so I see it every day. On it I have images of condos I want, places I want to go, and words and phrases that mean something to me and act as daily reminders of my goals. Even if I just glance in its direction, it's a subconscious reminder of what I really want out of my life.

GOAL BOOKS

As I mentioned, I do not look at my goal book daily or even weekly or monthly. I am lucky my head is attached or I would probably forget to bring it with me every morning as I am rushing to get the kids to school, so forget adding another task to my list! Still, there is a magical power that comes from articulating your goals with a pen and paper, even if you only visit it once a year. Maybe it's just the clarity we get from organizing our thoughts and desires which helps us to get a better plan of attack in place. But I can assure you taking the time to do these small activities will have a huge impact on your overall aspirations.

GOAL-SETTING TIPS

Remember, you will have different goals for different areas of your life. Personally, I divide my goal setting into these five areas:

- Family
- Career
- Health/fitness
- Social
- Spiritual

Notice the last one says "spiritual." This doesn't have to mean religion or church. To me spiritual is anything which fulfills your spirit and makes you happy. For example, it could be charity and/or philanthropic work, meditation or relaxation.

Always make goals specific and attached to a timeline. Saying "I want a million dollars" is great but by not having a clearly defined outcome or goal date, you are essentially just making a wish. A better approach would be to say "I want to build my business to make $1,000,000 net income annually in ten years" or let's say—for a fitness goal—"I want to lose five percent body fat over the next six months." Now, instead of just a statement, you have a clearly defined goal and then you can devise a strategic plan of action to achieve it. This is best done using a timeline to hold yourself accountable. Speaking of which…

You Are Not Five Years Old

Now that you have your goals outlined, let's talk about the next step in the process. BEING PRODUCTIVE! Goals are great but they become completely worthless if you don't do anything productive to work on them! This concept is where you really have to BYOB. You cannot be productive without having personal accountability and to do this you must put your #biggirlpantson.

PERSONAL ACCOUNTABILITY IS WHAT SEPARATES THE WINNERS FROM THE LOSERS.

It's what defines the people who achieve success and the people who talk shit. It's the bikini or the one piece! Your goals are going to take a lot of hard ass work—and no one else is going to do the work for you. You need to step up to the damn plate! You are not five years old. You do not have a babysitter following you around telling you what to do and smacking your butt if you don't do it. You need to realize right now your success is completely up to you. You have to practice keeping yourself productive and accountable until it becomes second nature; even then, it takes a lot of effort. Be prepared to put in the work.

Accomplishing anything of importance takes a ton of discipline, self-awareness and sacrifices. You may have to sacrifice your free time, your social routines, and even your comfort at times, but with any great sacrifice comes great reward. I can personally attest that sticking to your goals and holding yourself accountable is one of the greatest feelings of accomplishment a woman can have and is well worth every drop of blood, sweat, and tears you lose along the way. I will talk a lot more about productivity and time management in a later chapter but for now just let this sink in. ★

CHAPTER 2

Get Out of Your Way

AS YOU WERE reading chapter 1, you may have wondered why I'm talking so much about goals, personal accountability and the like. You deal with all these things at work but how do they affect your fitness? The reason is simple: Fitness is 100 percent mental. Ask any of the top fitness models or professionals you admire and each person will tell you the same thing. IF you cannot get you mind right, you will never get your body right. Period. It takes determination, will power, perseverance, grit, and an unrelenting commitment to consistency to achieve the body and life you desire. You need to be self- aware and always looking to improve. And, most importantly, remain open minded.

I am not going to sugar coat things like other trainers so you think all you have to do is buy a cool outfit and show up at the gym to get results. Screw that! Showing up at the gym is the easy part! It's the other twenty-three hours of the day you need to worry about; that's where you're going to struggle. Fitness is hard. I always joke that it's like that one really high maintenance friend who takes a lot of work, drains the crap out of you, and is sometimes really crazy—but for some reason you still love that bitch and you always find yourself back for more. You need to be mentally prepared for the work and realize you're going to hit road blocks and obstacles along the way, especially when you're trying to balance 5,467 things at one time. It's inevitable! And here is where most people go wrong: They are prepared for the physical work but disregard the mental work that's required to achieve real success and real LONG-Term results. The biggest obstacle you have to overcome isn't going to be surviving your workout; it's not going to be eating healthy, your schedule, your finances or your current fitness level or any other excuse I often hear. All of these things are completely manageable. The biggest, most pernicious obstacle you have to watch out for is the one that you least expect: YOUR MIND.

THE SILENT KILLER

When we are little, our parents tell us we can be anything we want when we grow up—astronauts, movie stars, firefighters, heck, even the president! We feel infallible. We let nothing inhibit our beliefs or intentions. We cannot be stopped!

And then we grow up.

Somehow along the path to adulthood we lose a lot of our confidence. We are told that we're stupid, can't pay attention, need to try harder and do better. Our ideas get laughed at. We fail, A LOT. Even more, the media barrages us as young girls with images of rail thin models and flawless movie stars on TV. We feel pressure to look like them, and if we don't we feel inferior and unworthy, we create unrealistic expectations in our heads and hold ourselves to these standards, which leads

to a snowball effect of low confidence and self-worth.

And for most of us this is it.

These beliefs and thoughts become deeply ingrained into our subconscious where they stay and affect us unknowingly for the rest of our lives. They become the silent killer that extinguishes every fire we have within ourselves to be better and do better; they act as sandbags around our feet, making it almost impossible to get anywhere we are trying to go. They are the sole reason we become our own worst critics. And until this internal dialogue is addressed, you will have a difficult time reaching your full potential in anything.

THE PINK SPONGE

I want you to do the following exercise with me for a minute:

Think about a pink dish sponge. Picture its rectangular shape, its bumpy and soft texture, and its bright pink color. Picture squirting soap on it as you begin to wash all of the dishes in your sink. And just as you begin to pour water on the sponge—making it all sudsy to wash them—STOP.

For the next sixty seconds I want you to totally forget about the pink sponge. Erase it from your mind completely! Impossible, right? No matter how hard you try to ignore or repress it, the thought of the pink sponge keeps creeping back in.

Negative thoughts act much the same way as the lingering impression of the sponge. No matter how hard you try to get rid of them, they become the sneaky little insecurities and fears which hold you back without you even knowing.

If you were lucky when you were growing up, you had parents who helped combat some of this damage by reinforcing your positive attributes and helping you to make sense of it all. However, most of you probably still have some of these negative thoughts or beliefs about yourself deep down inside influencing everything you do and say. In fact, this is the primary reason I was inspired to write this book.

GETTING RID OF YOUR SPONGE

What does success mean to you? For some, it's money or fame; for others, it is achievement. Regardless of your personal definition, becoming successful means reaching your full potential. To do this, people must have a positive inner dialogue and beliefs about themselves and their abilities. You've probably heard the cliché quote, "the first step to achieving is believing." In fact, this line is incredibly accurate on all counts. I will say this again: You have to get your mind right. You cannot have negative thoughts buried in your subconscious acting as a pink sponge and absorbing every ounce of positive energy you have. YOU NEED EVERY OUNCE OF THIS ENERGY TO WORK ON YOUR GOALS!

The first step to getting rid of your sponge is first acknowledging it's there. You have to become self- aware of your thoughts and actions to learn about yourself and recognize the patterns which hold you back. Now, I am not a psychologist or psychiatrist; however, I have been to a few through the years so I can speak firsthand about how profound the impact of addressing the pink sponge can be on your entire life. It affects everything from your personal relationships, friendships, business, and of course your health and wellness in ways you would never imagine. Although I can't diagnose or prescribe anything, I can tell you about my own experience and some of the things which helped me and a few other very successful people break free of our sponges. It has been, by far, my biggest personal achievement yet.

Growing up, I had been to a few psychiatrists for my "attention" issues so it wasn't an uncommon thing for me; but it wasn't until my most recent experience with a clinical psychologist where I made HUGE progress in becoming self-aware and breaking free from the confines of my sponge.

I am not going to get into my life-long story (lord knows that would be entertaining lol) but to summarize, some of the things I was dealing with at that time were the need for constant validation from others, self- doubt, feelings of selfishness related to being a busy mom/wife/daughter, marital issues, and more. The list was pretty long now that I think about it. For someone who looked as if she was all put together and had a perfect life on the outside, internally I was dealing with a ton of stress and anxiety which ultimately led me to become very sick and unhappy. It was time for a change.

I was referred to my therapist by a good friend who told me he uses a technique called "Eye Movement Desensitization and Reprocessing (EMDR)" and that I should try to talk to him about everything. I went in reluctantly, thinking I was too smart to be helped by some person who thinks he "understands" everyone. I remember I was very skeptical that these sessions would do anything, and especially annoyed because I didn't really "have the time" to go to them in the first place. Boy, was I wrong and I am so I thankful I went! It ended up being one of the best decisions I have ever made and I am so grateful that I took my friend's advice. More importantly, I was very happy I made the time.

Without getting into too much technical detail, EMDR is a technique which allows the therapist to bypass your conscious mind and access your subconscious mind and thoughts. Our subconscious mind is where we store all of our old memories and emotions; its where we bury and repress unpleasant or hurtful memories. It's our emotional mind, while conversely our conscious mind is our rational mind. They are like ying and yang.

After doing a few sessions, I was completely and utterly shocked at what I was holding on to! Until I went through this exercise, I never realized how powerful our subconscious mind is and how profoundly it affects us daily. Things that happened to us, even as children, remain there and then creep into our conscious mind and affect our thoughts without us knowing. Let me give you an example to which I know you can relate. Have you ever been so annoyed or repulsed by something but you have no idea why? Or had an unusually vehement reaction to someone or something over a seemingly minor issue? That is your subconscious at play. Small insignificant things act as "triggers" which make you react differently—and almost uncontrollably—because of some memory or emotion you have stored in your subconscious. I found out there were things I had absolutely no idea affected me in a very big way. In fact, I recall laughing at the first memory which popped up in my head during my first session because it seemed so silly. Well, after memory after memory kept popping up with the same underlying theme and issue I realized it did impact me, MUCH more than I could have ever imagined! Some of my characteristic behaviors and thought processes made sense after I realized some of the things I was harboring. And until we addressed these thoughts and emotions, they would continue to do so.

Learning how these memories affected me was enlightening to say the least and helped me to become extremely self-aware of my reactions and behaviors. It enabled me get over some of the feelings which were limiting me and my ability to reach my full potential in a lot of ways. I read a book years ago called *The Big Leap* and although I knew at that time I had been—as the author called it—"Upper Limiting," I had no idea why or how to fix it. Upper limiting, according to the author Gay Hendricks, is when people have some limiting beliefs and emotions which hold them back from achieving the next level of success, whether that is taking the next step in a career, going to the next level in a relationship, or even committing to health and fitness goals. If you have ANY kind of negative or false beliefs going on internally they will always work their way into your daily life and ruin any chance you have of progress. These thoughts and beliefs are your pink sponge.

If you're struggling to make progress—in any area of life—I strongly urge you to look into different techniques to help address some of these issues. This goes for both personal struggles (negative self- talk, insecurities, fear, personal goals) and interpersonal struggles (relationships, friendships, career). There are many other techniques so do some research and find out what's best for you. Working to identify and eliminate your pink sponge will be one of the best investments you can ever make and the Return on Investment (ROI) will be dramatic. The types of goals we're going after take as much energy and motivation as possible so it's imperative to have a positive mindset so you don't hold yourself back. Being self-aware and free of your sponge is instrumental to getting where you want to go when you want to get to the next level. And that is EXACTLY where we are going! ★

CHAPTER 3

The Secrets to Success

NOW THAT YOU have your goals and your mind is right, let's talk about the next step to becoming a Bikini Boss: ACTION! Now, I'm not just talking about any action; I'm talking about specific, focused, deliberate action. That's the kind of action that is going to help you build momentum *toward* your goals, not away from them.

It's easy to make goals and say you want to do something but the difficult part is getting those things done. Instant gratification makes it easy for us to get addicted to things which, in turn, make us want to do them more. We show up to work, we get paid; we drink coffee, we get a buzz; we post something online, we get likes. Fitness, on the other hand, works differently. Although you feel better right away, the physical and aesthetic results do not happen overnight. There is no instant gratification; it takes time, consistency, and perseverance. For this reason, you have to become really good at self-motivation and

avoiding procrastination like the plague.

Don't be fooled. I am writing about this because I am the QUEEN of procrastination. In fact, it took me forever to get all of this information into a book! My only saving grace is that I am very self-aware and I have become very good at managing my weaknesses. I have learned it is something I have to overcome if I want to achieve big things in life. Remember: you have to BYOB.

In order to have the time you need to achieve your fitness goals, you have to be as efficient and productive as possible. I am going to share a few of my most effective time management/productivity tactics for you to implement in your own life so you can have more time to get more important things done (like going to the gym).

GET ORGANIZED

There are some of you who are type A and already have your act together, and then there are some of you who cringe at the thought of taking the time to do so. Although I usually fall into the latter category, I have learned that taking time to get organized is incredibly beneficial. In fact, you would be surprised at the impact doing even small tasks such as cleaning out your purse, car, refrigerator, Tupperware cabinet, and closet can have on your sanity. I am not sure if it's the actual ACT of doing these things which stimulates our brain and in turn, makes us more clear minded, focused, and task oriented, or if it's the result of being more productive from spending less time shuffling through stuff trying to remember where we left that one important paper or our keys. I think for me, it's a combination of both. Whatever it is, it has a ripple effect across all areas of my life and allows my brain to better focus and improves my desire to continue getting things done. ANOTHER beneficial side effect I experience from getting organized is that doing one task to completion makes me crave doing it again and again. It becomes the catalyst to more action by creating IN-STANT GRATIFICATON. You know exactly what I am talking about, too. The same

kind of gratification you get when you see vacuum lines on a carpet or lawn mower lines after mowing the lawn. Its pure satisfaction—YOU NEED THIS. You need to keep the action momentum going strong. If your natural tendency is to be a disorganized mess, you have to overcome it and create new habits to propel you in the right direction. The key to results is action, and getting organized is a surefire way to get you on the right path.

PLAN YOUR WEEK

Now that you are getting organized, it's time to take it to the next level. I'm sure you've heard the cliché "failing to plan is planning to fail." This line may be overused but I assure you it's true. When you are juggling ten balls in the air it's a MUST you organize your week or else it's going to literally run you ragged. There are only so many hours in the day so you need to be smart and think through how you can organize your schedule to be as efficient as possible. Make sure you schedule times to go to the gym, to do housework, laundry, work, and playing with your kids, and whatever else is on your plate. Everything you have to do needs to be on that schedule and you must stick to it! You should also include time for personal growth such as meditation, reading, audiobooks, workshops, certifications, etc. You always need to work on your mind as well as your body. We will talk more about this in a later chapter.

Making a schedule is insanely important when it comes to having accountability for your actions because if you're not sticking to it you're going to feel guilty as hell and that little voice in your head will start telling you to focus. Conversely, without a schedule you have nothing to feel guilty about and therefore won't hold yourself accountable. Being proactive instead of reactive to life is key.

PLAN YOUR DAY

Every minute counts. If you want to reach your goals, you better act like it! Every morning on my way to work I think about everything I need to get done and give myself time parameters to do it. Mentally organizing your day will be another level of accountability, and lord knows we need as much as we can get! HERE IS ONE OF THE BEST TIPS I WILL GIVE YOU. If you take anything away from this chapter, make it this:

Every day I make an action list of the three most important things I need to get done. These are my top, most essential actionable items I must complete that day. If and when I get these items done, I will allot additional time for checking emails or completing ancillary tasks.

It's extremely easy to get distracted with "busy work," so make sure you know what your most important tasks are to move you toward your goals—and work on those like your life depends on it. This is where your big girl pants come in handy. You've got to hold yourself accountable to this list! Getting really good at this habit will change your life and subsequently allow you to change your body.

THE POWER OF LISTS

Call me crazy, but just as in writing down your goals, there is a lot of power in making task lists. Notice I didn't say "to-do" because it can be a list of things you need to buy or bring, etc. The same way getting organized activates your brain, making lists keeps those items in the forefront of your brain and also ensures you don't miss important stuff. This is especially important when you are trying to manage a million different things such as your kids' school events, work functions, and every other thing you need to stay on top of in your life. There are a ton of great apps available to use or—if you're like me—you can do it the old fashioned way and write it out yourself. My only recommendation is if you prefer to write out your lists make sure you keep them somewhere accessible where you can see it such as on a white board or a folder you use every day for work. Making a list is pointless if you never see it.

In addition to helping you remember everything, there is HUGE satisfaction which comes from checking items off your list. It's extremely motivating and will make you want to keep doing more and more, encouraging the same kind of activity you get from getting organized which will only keep propelling you towards your goals.

AIRPLANE MODE

You wake up, have your day all planned out, your task list on hand and you look at the clock—and before you know it, it's already five o'clock! You've gotten literally two things done on your list and now you're stressing because you have to add these items to tomorrow's list. Starting to sound familiar? With today's smart phones and extremely accessible Internet access to anyone and everyone around the world, in the blink of an eye, it's not surprising we have trouble staying focused! Work, work, text; work, work, email; work, work, update. … It's never ending. This is where you will have to work extremely hard to stay focused on the task at hand. It is certainly not easy; trust me I know this! BUT if you can master this you WILL reach your goals…or least get pretty damn close.

The struggle is real. My husband always makes fun of me because I get distracted so easily; I'm like the dog from the Disney movie *Up* when he sees another animal and starts chasing it… "Squirrel!" That's basically me all day every day—lol. I have learned the best way for me to manage this is by implementing what I have designated as "Airplane Mode": times where I click my phone into airplane mode so I don't get any calls, messages, emails or alerts. It's

hard to do sometimes, I'll admit, but I have found it to be one of the most effective productivity tactics I use and the only way I survive the constant barrage of communication which comes through my phone daily. If you have kids or anyone else you worry about having to reach you, I know what you're thinking (I am a crazy neurotic too!) but I can assure you it will be fine if you have your phone off for an hour or two. The sky isn't going to fall.

CONSISTENCY > PERFECTION

You've got your mind right, your big girl pants are on… you're chugging along, kicking life's ass when suddenly BAM! Life gives you a big ole bitch slap. Yes, I hate to tell you but shit will hit the fan at some point so you need to be prepared, mentally, to deal with it. Kids will get sick, people will not show up at work, you'll get sick, you'll have personal issues come up… that's all part of life. Understanding there will be times where you're rocking it and times where you're getting your ass kicked will be the difference between victory and defeat. Life can be tumultuous at times. Expect it. If you understand there are ups and downs, you can roll with the punches and jump back on when things calm down rather than throwing in the towel at the first little hiccup.

The best advice I can give you here is KEEP GOING. Things will get tough and you will want to quit at some point. I know this because I have been there and I still get there sometimes. Being successful isn't easy! Just because I look all put together doesn't mean I don't have moments of temporary insanity, because I do! The difference is I never allow myself to quit and I understand that no matter how crazy life gets, it will all calm down and get back to normal at some point and I keep going. One day you may get everything on your list done, plus some; the next, maybe only half. What matters most is that you keep the momentum going and you DO NOT QUIT! Understand, there is no such thing as perfect and consistency is the key. If you can drill this into your brain, you're on your way. ★

CHAPTER 4

Circle Getting Smaller

HERE IS WHAT most people don't talk about when it comes to your goals: you are going to face resistance.

It is an unfortunate fact that some people cannot be happy or supportive when other people are trying to better themselves and achieve their goals. This is a hard lesson to learn, and honestly, can be very hurtful, especially if it's coming from people you actually care about like your family and close friends. Be prepared, because you are going to make some people uncomfortable. They'll respond by trying to make you feel guilty about your ambitions and goals. It's all part of the process. Most people cannot do what you're doing; most people are friggin' lazy! They don't have the ambition, drive or grit to stick to anything so they try to bring you down to their level in order to feel better about themselves. This behavior is due completely to their insecurities and has absolutely nothing to do with you! You've got to understand this and realize they are simply projecting their own insecurities onto you because they are afraid to do it themselves. They don't have the balls. Period. I'm writing about this behavior because it's extremely prevalent in the fitness world. The second you commit to a better body and better health you're going to hear from people who call you obsessed, self-absorbed, selfish, and conceited. God forbid you post a fitness selfie—forget it! Women, of course, happen to be the absolute worst with this. It blows my mind when I hear about some of the things my clients have to deal with, and from their families nonetheless!

I believe this is an extremely important subject and one that other people rarely discuss in relation to success. I am here to prepare you for battle, the mental battle, that is.

You need to be aware of the traps, or as I prefer to call them "mind f**ks," these insecure people will use to try and sabotage your ambitions. Once you become aware, you can spot them from a mile away.

Let's take a minute and discuss the top mind f**ks you will hear from other people who have nothing better to do than trying to make you feel awful about working on yourself

MIND F**K #1
—YOU'RE SELFISH

This is my personal favorite and one that hits particularly close to home because some of my family and people I really cared about kept telling me this. Get this through your thick skull right now: YOU ARE NOT SELFISH! You deserve to take time to work on yourself. I don't care if you're a wife, girlfriend, daughter or mother. Everyone needs and deserves a little personal time. Whether it's taking time to go to the gym, going back to school, setting aside "mommy time" to do yoga or meditate, going for a massage, getting your nails done… you deserve these things! You should never feel guilty about taking time for yourself. Women, especially mothers, often put everyone else first. This is not a good habit. If you don't take the time to work on yourself, I can PROMISE you will end up resenting someone or something. Whether it be your job, your husband or even your mother, you will ultimately end up in a bad

situation if you cannot have five seconds to focus on yourself.

MIND F**K #2
—YOU'RE OBSESSED

Eyeroll. This one always makes me laugh. There is a big difference between being passionate about something and being obsessed. And quite frankly, if your "obsession" is something healthy which makes you feel amazing and confident, then what is wrong with that? NOTHING! When you start living this lifestyle, getting fit and feeling amazing, the results become addictive. When you understand you can look and feel the way you've always wanted, why would you want anything else! It's just like when people say you get "addicted" by going to the chiropractor; you don't get addicted; the problem is you realize how you SHOULD be feeling and moving so the second you feel differently, you are miserable. People who are unhealthy, uneducated or lazy will not understand this concept. They have no idea how it is to feel strong, healthy, energetic, and confident. They are used to feeling like garbage. Remember who you are dealing with and don't let their small-minded words bother you.

MIND F**K #3
—YOU'RE SELF-ABSORBED

Let's get this straight right now. THE ONLY PEOPLE WHO SAY THINGS LIKE THIS ARE

THE PEOPLE WHO ARE SELF-ABSORBED THEMSELVES! In psychology this is called projection. They feel this way about themselves, so they try to project it onto other people. There are a ton of people who do this quite frequently. But once you're aware of this tendency, you'll quickly learn not to take things personally because you don't have an issue—the other people have one. Deep down they are the ones who are self-absorbed so they can't stand to see someone else succeeding or doing better than them. These people are the same ones who will say you always talk about yourself or you only care about yourself, that you're conceited; meanwhile you go above and beyond to try to make them feel better all to realize it's completely futile because you will never make them happy. The real problem is they are not happy with themselves. Truly confident and secure people will never say things like this. They will be supportive and become your biggest fans! If anyone tells you something like this, EVER, run for the hills. You do not need that kind of negative energy in your life.

FOCUS ON YOUR OWN SHIT

Climbing the ladder to success is not easy. Ask people who have accomplished anything in life and they will tell you the same thing. You're going to get resistance from the people you least expect, sometimes even those whom you care about the most. Does it hurt? Hell yes, but you have to keep going. You can't let someone else's issues destroy your ambitions and dreams. You've worked way too hard for that! Stay focused, ignore the chirping, and focus on yourself and you'll be on your way. ★

Nadine Phillip >>

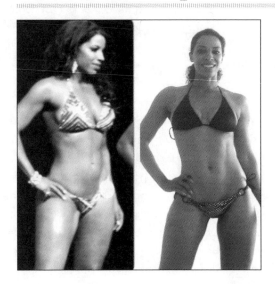

Age 35, Sr. Enterprise Account Executive

Started Training at age 32

Favorite happy meal: curry chicken roti ("I'm a true Trini gal at heart")

"No matter what is happening in your life you know that your health is not a concern. In fact, it is 100 percent within your control and constantly improving... workouts make me feel like I did something amazing for me!"

Nadine's Story: "How did I end up here?!" Haven't we all asked ourselves that at some point? At age 31, I found myself highly successful with a career in tech sales and booming little side business about to blow up.

I was on a business trip in the summer of 2011 when I just happened to step on a scale. I was curious . . . simply curious. I knew I had gained a little weight, because let's face it—balancing it all left little time for cooking and taking care of myself. But, even still, I wasn't feeling insecure about my body. When I looked down and saw the number I almost fell over. 172. One Hundred Seventy-Two. I stand 5'2". When did I stop being "little"? I went and got a tape measure . . . my hips were 49 inches. I could not believe my eyes!

And so my secret mission began. I didn't want anyone to know. I didn't want to have to ever admit that I lost control over my body while trying to maintain control over my life, so I set a goal and quietly began following a meal plan I found on a supplement box. I dusted off my L.L. Cool J

Platinum Work Out book (I got it as a gift mainly for the pictures) and I started lifting weights.

The thing is that this whole time I WAS working out. I was going to the gym five days a week to do cardio and I was going to yoga two to three times a week. I didn't understand that eating very little did not make a good diet.

I started my mission the first week of July and by mid-August I had lost 20 pounds. Imagine that… increasing my meals to five times a day and lifting weights and my body was singing! Feeling a little less timid about having to undergo a "transformation" I mentioned to my business partner that I wanted to compete in a fitness show. Within days, she had sent me a list of prep coaches that were highly reputable and I picked a show to train for. My next journey began.

I have Crohn's disease and didn't fully understand the importance of the macronutrient numbers of my food which I was told to follow which made my first competition prep hard. I didn't ask questions, I just stuck to my plan. I dropped from 150 pounds to 120 between September 1 and Christmas. My hips were down to 32 inches but I was completely unhealthy, moody, and constantly having flair ups with my Crohn's. I pushed through . . . 100 percent on plan and competed! Although I felt really lousy, I loved the stage so much I signed right back up and did it all over again. But something happened with me the second time around. I started to play with my diet myself. I used my coach's meal plan as recommendations and not "bible" and I was still off kilter and struggling with my health and flare-ups. And then I met Theresa.

We talked for hours about metabolic damage, naturopathic medicine, and nutrition. Committing to this as a lifestyle isn't feasible when you are on an extreme program—and my priorities had shifted significantly. I wasn't trying to lose weight anymore; I wanted to be healthy and continue to improve my physique. The more I learned about Theresa's health- and science-based program, the more confident I felt I would never be over-weight again. Let me repeat that: I would never be overweight again. Educating the clients about their health is the priority of the Bikini Boss Chicks program. To me, it's changed my life.

I signed up and haven't looked back. Working with Bikini Boss Chicks has provided me with a new sense of confidence that has changed the game for me. The difference? A coaching team that explains the program, the science and formula behind the custom meal plans and how they work with specific supplements for my body, has positioned me to take control over my body. Working with a team of brilliant, dedicated and supportive women has set my world on fire. The wit is quick, the support is fierce and the love is real. I would not recommend anyone else.

Nadine Phillips
Instagram @Deanierunn

Get in the Skinny

CHAPTER 5

That's Billion with a B

IF YOU'RE LIKE me, I'll bet the first thing that comes to mind when I say the words "diet industry" is an image of the Weight Watchers commercials or Jenny Craig from the 90s, or maybe Nutrisystem with its celebrity-laden endorsements. I could probably list a few more, too. And while you and I both know these are NOT the type of programs to follow if you want the body and results we are after, so many people think they are. Why is this?

If you grew up in the U.S, mostly likely you watched your mom or grandmother do Jane Fonda workout videos and take step aerobics classes. You've probably heard them talking about low calorie, low fat, low sugar, low carb, Atkins, Juice cleanse, ideal protein, high protein, no protein...are these starting to ring a bell? If there is a diet, they've probably tried it; and they are not alone. There is a reason for this! The diet industry is a $20 billion industry. The diet companies are GREAT at creating repeat customers, the ones who come ready to buy hundreds if not thousands, of dollars' worth of products or services. Understanding how and why they are able to do this is the key to unlocking your own long-term results and it all has to do with a shift in your paradigm.

"PARADIGM: a distinct set of concepts or thought patterns, including theories, methods, postulates, and standards for what constitutes legitimate contributions to a field."

Looking at the paradigm of the diet and fitness industry over the last forty years, it's easy to understand HOW the companies are able to create such a large market for new products and services and a plethora of eager consumers waiting to buy the latest quick fix program or fad diet plan. *That's what the old paradigm is designed to do.* You see, until relatively recently, it was thought the most effective way to get in shape was to use the "calories in, calories out" approach. The less you ate, the more you burned, the better you were. Everything became about losing weight, counting calories, and endless cardio. Gyms popped up everywhere with packed schedules of aerobics classes and filled with lines of treadmills and steppers for dieters to "burn" off what they ate. TV, radio, magazines, and newspapers touted the latest and greatest weight loss products. There were pills to make you not eat, pills to make you pee a lot, pre-packaged foods, exercise gimmicks; you name it, they made it. It didn't matter how many products or programs were released; there were always consumers enthusiastically waiting to buy. It was the perfect scenario, but not for the consumer.

THE VICIOUS CYCLE

Ebb and flow, up and down, back and forth; in the diet world we refer to this state of affairs as "yo-yo" dieting. Not surprisingly, it's pretty much the unfortunate reality for virtually all the people who have or are still trying to reach their weight loss goals. This constant state of weight gain and weight loss is a side effect of the old paradigm and for one reason only: the goal with the old paradigm is to lose weight. The goal is not to increase one's metabolism or stimulate fat burning hormones; it's not to build lean muscle or burn fat. The goal is to lose weight, period. Let me explain the myth of the yo-yo dieting epidemic.

In order to effectively lose weight, you must drastically cut calories and/or increase caloric expenditure at the same time. Is this feasible? Yes, absolutely. Whether it is sustainable is the question we should really be asking. It is one thing to cut calories and increase energy output for a few weeks; it is another thing to do it over the long term. Long term weight loss diets usually fail because there are three fundamental problems with this approach:

First, while you're dieting and restricting calories, you're losing weight, some of which is muscle, fat and some water. But what do you think happens once you resume a somewhat normal diet again? Exactly, you gain it all back! That's because weight loss diets are extremely taxing on the body. When you're dieting, your body is not getting the calories and nutrients it needs to run properly. As a result, the body has to get its energy from somewhere else so it starts to break down non-carbohydrate sources in the body to use as fuel in a process called gluconeogenesis. You would think this is ideal. However, the body is not only attacking fat; when the body is deficient of calories for prolonged periods, it utilizes other sources such as amino acids as well. Amino acids are the building blocks of protein in the body. When your body needs to utilize amino acids for energy, it will efficiently attack places where large amounts of protein are stored such as your skeletal muscle. Muscle is your friend. It's your metabolic machine that burns fat and calories while you're at rest; you cannot afford to lose it! The key to getting a toned lean body is having lean muscle and using food and exercise to speed up your metabolism not slow it down. The key to LONG-Term results is having a strong metabolic machine. Starving yourself will destroy your metabolic machine; starving yourself is NOT the answer.

Secondly, it is extremely unhealthy, both mentally and physically, to deprive yourself for long periods of time. Being involved in the competitive fitness industry I have seen how deprivation diets affects girls and can cause all kinds of problems; including serious eating disorders. There is a big difference between discipline and deprivation. Discipline is having the willpower to make good choices and eat foods which will give your body the nutrients necessary to achieve your goals. Deprivation is restricting yourself from major food groups, like carbs or fats, and eating very low calorie diets for long periods of time. Deprivation is starvation and deprivation is extreme. Our bodies are designed to have balance and equilibrium and avoid extremes at all cost. And just like a thermostat, we have settings built in to automatically keep our body and physiology at specific conditions for optimal health.

Homeostasis: *the property of a system in which variables are regulated so that internal conditions remain stable and relatively constant.*

In layman's terms, this process called homeostasis is an innate mechanism built in to our genes to protect the body from extreme conditions which could greatly affect our survival rate. Extreme conditions such as temperature change, PH conditions and starvation which would greatly affect ur survival rate. OUR BODIES ARE DESIGNED TO SURVIVE. They will fight us tooth-and-nail to avoid going into gluconeogenesis by adapting our neurological hormones and brain pathways to make us seek and attain food. And, trust me, our bodies will win. Messing with your thermostat is extremely dangerous and unhealthy and a gateway for addictions. If you think you can't get addicted to food, think again. Food addiction is a legitimate illness. Just as with a drug addict or alcoholic, you are creating an environment in which your brain chemistry changes and creates a subsequent behavioral issue. Deprivation diets are a sure fire recipe for physiological chaos and should be avoided at all costs. They are not a sustainable approach.

THAT'S BILLION WITH A B

Lastly, extreme diets and excessive exercise take a huge toll on the adrenal glands by creating a stress response in the body. This leads to a range of negative metabolic effects, ultimately affecting your hormones and leaving you in a poor metabolic state. Even worse, left unchecked, this physiological stress can lead to a vast array of health problems. It's much more serious than you probably realize and new research on the importance of metabolic health is coming out every day. This is such an important topic I am going to actually discuss in detail how stress affects us in chapter 7 but for now I want to emphasize that deprivation diets create a massive stress response in the body which is devastating for both your fat-loss goals and your overall health and well-being. ★

CHAPTER 6

Myths of the Old Paradigm

IN THE LAST chapter we learned that the old paradigm is based off the desired outcome of weight loss and the fundamental problems with this approach. Regardless of the overwhelming evidence, science and research available today, so many people are still caught up in this old paradigm and its belief system.

In any industry, there is a very small sector of people who stay up on the latest news, trends, research, etc.; the majority of the consumers do not. We call this minority the "early adopters." They're the people who are obsessed with and/or consumed with that particular area, product or subject. The early adopters are the ones who pass the latest trends, research and information along to the majority. The majority of people are the laggards, the ones who are extremely slow or the last to learn or adapt.

I am an early adopter. I eat, sleep and breathe fitness and nutrition, and I have done so for the past twelve years. It's my job to research and learn the most up-to-date and effective information and science possible for myself and my clients. Most people do not have the time and/or energy to spend learning, researching and applying this information, or more likely, they don't really care to. Consequently, when it comes time to "get in shape," they fall back on what they know—the status quo. You probably were in this group at some point, but if you're reading this book you are moving from the end of the laggards' line, closer to the early adaptors. Kudos to you!

Now that you're starting to understand the truth about health and fitness more clearly, I want to take a few minutes to debunk a few of the biggest myths perpetuated by the old paradigm because these false beliefs are the very things keeping many women from having the body of their dreams. I want you to read and re-read these next few concepts until they become ingrained within you. Understanding these principles will be integral to your success with my program.

MYTH #1—
CARBS ARE EVIL

There is a huge misconception in the fitness industry that carbs are terrible and you cannot eat them if you want to see results. This could not be farther from the truth. Every week I get clients who have major carb sensitivity and/or metabolic damage from having been on super low carb diets for extended periods of time coupled with excessive exercise and/or cardio sessions. It's unnecessary and frankly just stupid. Now, I am not saying that you can't utilize short-duration, low-carb periods to your advantage because there can be huge benefits to Cyclical Ketogenic Diets (CKD) and modified carb cycling plans but only for certain desired outcomes and certain types of clients and NOT for prolonged periods of time. If you're a lifestyle client or four months before a show and your coach has you on an extended low carb plan, I would consider re-evaluating your strategy and long-term goals. You will probably see rapid results, but the effect on your metabolism isn't worth it.

Dr. Atkins had brilliant marketing and branding strategies and managed to successfully brainwash everyone into believing that carbs are evil and must be avoided at all costs. But we now know that this is absolutely NOT the case. The goal with any nutrition program should be to keep the client healthy and get results without restricting any macro nutrient food group for an extended amount of time. This also applies to other macro-nutrients like fat and protein; low fat diets are not healthy either! The body works all together as one big intricate system and trying to shortcut the system by drastic measures will cause a malfunction in the long run.

Carbs such as potatoes, rice, fruit, etc. are not essential for survival but are necessary if you're trying to get the results and look you desire with your physique. Understanding how much and when to take them is the key and we will be teaching you all of that in part three of this book.

MYTH #2—
YOU HAVE TO BE 100 PERCENT PERFECT AT ALL TIMES TO GET RESULTS

The biggest problem I see with clients is their all-or-nothing mentality. Do I eat perfectly clean and stay completely on track at all times? Hell no! I just ate kettle chips last night. If you think that you have to be absolutely perfect at all times, the first time you have a slip up you will give up and quit because you "blew it." Then what? You fall right back into the trap of eating poorly, missing workouts, and feeling terrible. Screw that! That's exhausting.

REPEAT AFTER ME: This is a lifestyle, NOT a diet.

You have to be realistic and have the right mindset to achieve the body you want and maintain long-term results. We are not following a "diet" like the old paradigm. We are eating to fuel our body and to optimize our metabolism. If you shift your paradigm and way of thinking you will understand it's not about perfection; it's about CONSISTENCY.

A sound goal we use at Bikini Boss Fitness is the 80/20 rule. Eighty percent of the time we eat to fuel our body and make smart choices to give it the nutrients it needs to run properly. Twenty percent of the time we eat for enjoyment. Food is an integral part of our social and cultural traditions. You need to have some flexibility to be able to enjoy these occasions without guilt or remorse. Remember from the last chapter, deprivation is not healthy for your mind or body and making yourself avoid indulgences at all costs will have a massive backlash. Balance and moderation are paramount for the success of our clients.

MYTH #3—
YOU MUST STARVE YOURSELF TO GET RESULTS

If I had to give only one piece of advice to help you transform your physique it would be to fuel your body. As a coach, I often meet women who cannot fathom the idea they need to eat frequently… and eat a lot! In fact, this is probably the most prevalent issue I see when women start training with me. Due to the old paradigm, you would assume a lack of results is due to over consumption; however, it's almost always from eating too little or eating the wrong type of food. News flash: I eat more than most men! So do all of my clients and the thousands of other Bikini Fitness models whom you aspire to look like. If you look at me you probably wouldn't think so because we are conditioned to think if a woman is in shape she must be starving herself but I'm here to tell you that is absolutely not the case. It's just the opposite, actually. You have to give your body what it needs to make changes or it won't change—end of story.

No nutrients = no change.

Think about this for a second—would you expect a race car to win a race running on fumes? No. It needs gasoline to run! Just like cars need gasoline, our body needs nutrients from food. Nutrients are what our body uses to run properly; that includes the food we eat, water we drink, and supplements we take. They are the building blocks to our metabolism. If you think I'm crazy right now, telling you to eat MORE food, take a look at the people you know on a low calorie "weight loss" diet and ask yourself whether you want to look like them. They may be smaller but they are soft and flabby with no tone or definition anywhere. Trust me when I tell you, your nutrition is integral to your success. You can have the best workout from the best trainer and still not get results. It all comes down to your diet.

MYTH #4—
IT'S AN OVERNIGHT PROCESS

Get out of the old paradigm! This is not a quick fix solution. We are conditioning our metabolisms and building our bodies to run like a metabolic machine. This takes time. If it took you six months or six years to put the weight on, it's certainly not going to come off in two weeks. You have to be realistic with your goals and what it's going to take to achieve them or you are setting yourself up for failure before you even begin. Weight loss is easy. You stop eating, you work out more, and you lose weight. But we already know this is NOT the answer to your problems. We know this is NOT a sustainable long-term solution and we know this is NOT what you want to look like. This type of thinking will not get you to your goals. You need to align your thinking

with your goals to reach success. If you follow any Bikini Fitness models, you will see it takes months and sometimes years for them to go through their transformations. So, stop expecting yours to be overnight. This is a marathon, not a race. Only the patient survive.

MYTH #5—
THE SCALE IS THE ONLY MEASURE OF SUCCESS

This is the biggest, most detrimental myth of them all. THE SCALE DOES NOT MATTER! We are NOT trying to lose weight. We are trying to speed up your metabolism and turn your body into a fat burning machine. In order to do this, we need to use food and exercise to build lean muscle. Muscle is much denser than fat; it takes up less volume, ounce for ounce, than fat. Are you getting the point here? Yes, some people may lose weight on this program because everyone's metabolism is different. If you're starting off obese, meaning you have body fat which is thirty percent and higher, you are more likely to lose weight than a person who is skinny fat with no muscle. Take me, for example. I am 5'10'. I used to weight 135—140 pounds MAX. I ate like a bird, did cardio non-stop, and guess what? I HATED my body. I was perpetually frustrated with the results I was getting from all of the work I was putting in. I had it all wrong! I was stuck in the old paradigm. It wasn't until I learned HOW to properly eat and train for my goals that I saw the results I wanted and was truly happy and confident. And guess what else? I gained fifteen pounds! I now weigh the most I have ever weighed and I am the most happy with my body. I could have never gotten here had I been fixated only on losing weight.

Stop looking to the scale for results! You will know whether the program is working or not. You will feel better, your clothes will be looser, everything will start to tighten up, and your friends will comment on how good you look. But most importantly, you will feel better than you have in a long time. THAT is how we measure success, not by some meaningless numbers. Focus on being healthy and feeling good. Focus on creating habits that allow you to make this your lifestyle and get out of the toxic vicious cycle. I promise, if you commit to this type of thinking, the results will come before you know it. As I mentioned before, I am not the type to sugarcoat reality. I want you to understand the truth and what it takes. I want you to be successful! There is no magic wand or quick fix that will give you results which actually last. It takes a lot of work, hard ass work, but it will pay off. If you're looking for a quick fix or simply to lose weight you've already failed. ★

CHAPTER 7

You can't Run from Stress

STRESS LESS. I know this may seem impossible for some of you but I want to take a second and talk about what stress actually does to our bodies, on a physiological level, because it is SO IMPORTANT in regards to optimal fat loss physiology and overall health. The word "stress" can be used to describe anything that creates a stress response in the body, meaning it triggers an adrenal response causing

excess cortisol to be released, leading to a cascade of negative effects which I will discuss below in a minute. Our body can interpret stress from many sources; it can be physical stress, emotional stress, physiological stress, mental stress, and so on. Every negative thought, poor dietary choice, lost hour of sleep, and the typical daily grind all create stress on the body leading to an undesirable hormonal response and ultimately the degradation of tissues and storing of fat. This intrinsic hormonal response is so devastating to fat loss physiology, I want to make sure you understand the importance

of getting it under control before you even attempt to start any kind of program.

THE ANATOMY OF A STRESS RESPONSE

Now remember, a *stressor* is anything that creates a stress response in the body. It can be your negative thoughts, other people, driving in traffic, eating too much or too little, not sleeping enough, not loving your job, your boss and so on…. All of these things ultimately have the same effect on your body and it's not a positive one. Let's take a look at what this actually looks like on a physiological level:

A stressor is present -> your adrenal glands release excess cortisol to prepare your body to "fight or flight" -> the hormones tell your body to stop digesting food and shunt blood from your internal organs to your arms and legs (so we can fight or run away) -> the excess cortisol simultaneously signals the body to increase your blood sugar to make sure you have energy to fight or run away.

This hormonal process is a completely natural and healthy response which evolved back in the Paleolithic days to keep us alive as we encountered large beasts and had to hunt and scavenge for our food. Today, if we still needed to fight or run for our lives there would be no issues and the body would resume its normal physiology after the stressor was gone and we would continue life as usual. No big deal. Again, this is a NORMAL and healthy response to stress; there is nothing wrong with our bodies reacting this way. However, this innate response began to become a negative when we started being bombarded by chronic stress as is prevalent today. Essentially, our bodies cannot tell the difference between the stress from the proverbial saber tooth tiger or just a bad day at work.

So what happens if we don't need to fight or sprint away and the stress is just an ongoing daily occurrence? Well, remember, the ultimate goal of this hormonal response is to make sure we have enough energy to fight or run for our lives. It's a survival mechanism and to survive we need energy. Our body goes through all of these processes to ultimately surge a ton of sugar into the blood. If there's no tiger and no hunt, the extra energy isn't necessary. The excess blood sugar stays unused, floating around in our blood causing a ton of inflammation, damaging our tissues and organs, and disrupting our metabolic hormones. It ends up being stored in our insulin sensitive tissues, predominately around the belly. If this weren't bad enough, since you are not digesting your food properly, that too ends up rotting in your organs and creates all kinds of gut imbalances like bloating, gas, and leaky gut syndrome to name a few. These gut disturbances ultimately lead to massive nutrient deficiencies. It's a slippery slope of negative results which keeps snowballing. Keep the stressors present long term and your body will eventually think it is starving and will start using its own muscle for sugar as discussed previously, wasting it away and destroying your metabolic machinery. Kept ongoing, this will lead to a complete metabolic catastrophe in no time.

What I have just described is really only the tip of the iceberg. This stress response, if left unchecked, can lead to Metabolic Syndrome X, diabetes and a host of other stress induced diseases. While I do understand it's impossible to completely avoid stress, my goal here is to educate you on its causes and effects so you will have a better understanding and awareness and can learn how to minimize the stress in your life.

As you will find out in the next few chapters, muscle is the foundation of your metabolic machine so you will need to do everything possible to avoid wasting it. Supplements, sleep, proper diet, and exercise will help a great deal to mitigate this response but you still need to be aware of its effects from people, relationships, and other things with which I cannot help you. Stress is ultimately not good for your desired body or your health. ★

CHAPTER 8

Metabolism 101

IF YOU FOLLOW me on social media you know that nutrition is something I am insanely passionate about because it has changed my body and my life in a huge way. It is one of my favorite topics to research and discuss and I have spent years studying and applying different principles—with myself and my clients—to find out the best way to shred fat, build muscle, and, most importantly, stay healthy.

WHAT IS MY PHILOSOPHY ON NUTRITION AND SUPPLEMENTATION?

There are so many different objectives for "getting in shape." What is ideal for health is not always ideal for fat loss and vice versa. My philosophy about health and nutrition has always been to use the HEALTH-IEST approach to fat loss possible; using diet, exercise and supplements to speed up the metabolism, increase lean muscle and accelerate fat loss. I have learned that while some of the "quick fix" methods and programs out there do produce results, they are almost always short lived and often do much more damage than you think. *The good news is you don't need quick fix or extreme diets to get results.* With the proper knowledge and guidance you can get the body of your dreams and feel absolutely amazing without sacrificing your metabolism or your health. Not only have I done it with all my clients, I've done it myself and I am going to explain to you one of the pillars of my programs in this chapter.

There are no FDC approved supplements. The safest and most effective supplements are made from an FDA approved lab. As with any diet or exercise program, always consult your physician first.

WHY ARE SUPPLEMENTS SO IMPORTANT?

Some people say you don't need supplements if you eat healthy whole foods. But that is simply not true! Now, I'm not saying it's not important to eat a healthy, balanced diet of real whole foods, because it absolutely is, but there are many reasons you NEED to supplement with certain nutrients. Supplements are necessary, even if you have a healthy diet, for your fitness goals as well as your overall well-being.

First, in terms of nutrition, the food we produce today is nowhere near the quality of foods we used to eat. Between soil degradation, GMOs, and tons of chemicals and pesticides, food has lost much of its nutritional value and, in certain instances, actually works to leech nutrients from our bodies.

In response to what I've just said, you may be asking: But what about organic? Yes, I absolutely encourage you to purchase organic and non-GMO foods when possible. Unfortunately, there aren't many governing bodies inspecting "organic" farms so we have to trust that farmers are following the organic foods farming guidelines and standards. I hate to be a pessimist but in business most people are out to make a buck and will cut corners at all costs, especially if no one is looking.

If we don't know the quality of our food we cannot be sure we are giving our body what it needs to work properly. This is just one of the reasons I highly recommend taking a number of different supplements to make sure your body has all the vitamins and minerals it needs to function and run your metabolism properly.

Secondly, let's go back to STRESS again for a moment. We all have stress and much more than you are aware! Our current lifestyles are extremely demanding and our bodies take the brunt of it. Stress is the underlying factor which can make a healthy person's metabolism go haywire and yet, it's so often overlooked. I am going to explain, in great detail, just how it affects you and your metabolic potential.

We learned in the previous chapter that it doesn't matter whether it's physical, emotional or physiological stress, our bodies interpret it all the same exact way: A STRESSOR! In addition to our everyday stresses, training the way we do is not exactly the most natural thing to do to our bodies either. Even though our genes haven't changed since they evolved 50,000 years ago when we were hunters and gatherers living in caves the one thing that definitely HAS changed was our lifestyles. For example, you didn't see cave

44

women doing marathons and running around lifting weights and doing bikini contests. Humans at that time rarely took part in what we consider "exercise" and when they did it was either walking for long periods or super short, high intensity bursts of energy followed by long rest periods. This is how our bodies are genetically DESIGNED to move and understanding this concept is the key to boosting your metabolism

While physical exercise is absolutely healthy and essential, the type of training necessary to get a lean and toned look (like a Bikini Fitness model) actually can be stressful to our bodies if we don't take care of it and do the right thing. The right thing, in this instance, is taking precautionary measures to make sure our body has all of the nutrients it needs to function properly and produce results, without causing metabolic damage. Let's take a look at why:

METABOLISM 101:
Our bodies are one big
chemical reaction.
A + B = C

What do you think happens if you don't have B in the equation? Exactly, you don't get C! For purposes of your metabolism, "B" refers to vitamins, minerals, proteins, enzymes… these nutrients act as catalysts and are the foundation of your metabolism. They determine whether it's going to run like a souped-up Ferrari or an out-of-gas 1980s

Pinto with a dead battery. And we both know we definitely don't want the latter.

SO HOW DO WE AVOID THIS?

We already know our food quality is far from ideal and stress depletes our bodies of all the key nutrients necessary for our metabolisms to run efficiently. But let's take a closer look at the impact stress actually has on our body so that you'll understand exactly WHY supplementation is so critical for metabolic health….

RAWR! You're a cave woman just walking along the river looking for fish and out jumps a saber-toothed tiger! Your body immediately goes into a fight-or-fight response and starts operating to give you enough energy to fight this crazy beast or run for your life. Your adrenal glands start pumping, setting off a cascade of hormonal events that actually signal your body to stop digesting food and shunt blood from the intestines to your arms and legs because you need your extremities to have as much energy as possible. Next, it floods the body with blood sugar, making sure it has a constant source of fuel and subsequently immobilizing all of your metabolic functions because your primary focus is to fight the tiger or get the hell out of there!

Fast-forward 50,000 years. Today, we aren't running from saber-toothed tigers but we are under daily and sometimes hourly CHRONIC stress. And remember, our bodies interpret ALL stress the same way. Whether it's running from a saber-toothed tiger or just being annoyed at a slow driver, our annoying boss, unruly kids (or husbands) and so on… our adrenals are still operating the same way: HIGH GEAR. This wears our bodies down and, as you learned, totally disrupts our metabolic functions. To make the situation worse, what do you think happens when your body shunts blood to your limbs and stops digesting food? Your body stops getting the nutrients it needs to run properly.

Poor digestion = poor nutrition = deficiency = metabolic catastrophe

Not only are you not getting the nutrients you need, the partially digested food is now rotting in your gut which can cause a TON of problems in itself—including leaky gut and systemic inflammation to name just two. You can easily see how this process depletes us of essential nutrients and, if left unchecked, can ultimately lead to massive metabolic damage. And, trust me, I've seen it over and over again! Along with my husband who is a wellness physician, I previously owned and operated two health clubs where we specialized in metabolic damage. Through the programs we ran, I was able to work with hundreds of clients, both in person and online, all of whom had some form of metabolic damage. The problems could all be attributed to one thing: NUTRIENT DEFICIENCY.

THIS IS WHERE SUPPLEMENTS COME IN

The best way to ensure your body has what it needs to function at its highest level physiologically is to take certain supplements we KNOW our body needs to function metabolically. As I explain to my clients, there is no point even starting a fat loss program if you're not first making sure your body has what it needs to even burn fat! Trying to supercharge your metabolism and burn fat without the right nutrients is like trying to win a NASCAR race with an empty tank of gas; it's just not going to happen. As we saw in our chemistry lesson earlier, if we are missing key nutrients necessary for our bodies to work properly—it won't. End of story. It's not physiologically possible. There are certain supplements essential for health, some essential for fat loss and others needed for sports performance. Since health is the foundation of the latter two, I'm going to start with the fundamentals and discuss them all respectively.

YOU ARE WHAT YOU EAT—LITERALLY.

One of the best investments you can make for your health and fitness is in the quality of food and supplements you consume. This is not an area I would recommend being a cheapskate. Products that are dirt cheap are that way for a reason. Whether it's chicken breast or glutamine, you cannot mass produce a quality product cheaply. Keeping prices low at a grand scale means there are shortcuts taken in the production process to help increase profit margins. If you don't think companies would do this, you are being extremely naïve. When you have been in the health and fitness industry as long as I have, you learn quickly there are thousands of supplement companies claiming their products are superior but only a few can actually back up these claims. Many manufacturers cut corners and use fillers and different ingredients than what is stated on the label to increase profit margins and drive sales. Considering you are putting these substances in your body you always, ALWAYS need to do your research and make sure they are legitimate products. For supplements, a good rule of thumb is to stick with products made in FDA approved labs. While the FDA does not approve the actual supplements themselves, they do inspect and approve the facilities used to produce the supplements. Using a company which makes its products in an FDA approved lab—the label will say if it is—will ensure the product was tested to make sure only the key ingredients are in there and nothing else is. It's the best form of quality control you can get and worth the extra few bucks when you purchase your supplements.

I will now discuss the top five supplements I recommend to my clients and explain how and why they are integral to your metabolism.

1. MULTIVITAMIN: We understand our bodies are like a big chemical reaction, requiring and using different nutrients to get a desired metabolic result. But if we aren't getting the ideal amount of nutrients from food and our digestion is frequently impaired due to stressors, how do you expect our metabolisms to preform optimally? Exactly, they won't! This's why it's critical to take a quality multivitamin to make sure your body has what it needs to run efficiently. IT'S THE FOUNDATION OF YOUR METABOLISM. If you only had the money to purchase one supplement, I would tell you this is the one you should take. Remember, our goal is to win the NASCAR race; we need to have gas in our tank before we can start supercharging the engine. Quality is of utmost importance here. As any supplement expert can explain, it's very difficult to press a ton of different ingredients into one little block which is why it's best to look for brands that use capsule form. If you pick up the bottle, shake it and it sounds like rocks, put it back down and walk away. Your body isn't going to be able to digest them effectively and you'll be wasting your money. Secondly, look for a nutraceutical multivitamin formula. Nutraceutical vitamins contain additional nutrients like antioxidants and enzymes for maximal health benefits, plus they're usually chelated for better absorption. (Chelated means firmly attached, usually to an amino acid or other organic component, so the two don't separate during digestion.)

2. OMEGA-3 FISH OR KRILL OIL: Omega-3 fats are critical for health and are used to make every single cell in our bodies. When I say every single cell, I'm being literal—your hair, nails, skin, nerve, organs, and muscle. Our bodies are always in demand of omega-3 fats. Most people's diets are generally deficient in omega-3 and high in omega-6 and omega-9 which can cause inflammation, so it's not only essential but critical to supplement with omega-3 to bring back proper balance and regulate your hormones. Personally, when making my client's meal plans, I include omega-3 fats as at least one or two servings of liquid fat per day. You absolutely cannot overdose; it's not a pharmaceutical, it's a fat. If you're deficient in Omega-3 fatty acids, your body is going to use the little bit that you have for your brain and nerve cells. This is not good because all the other tissues, like muscle cells, will be deficient. *Why is this important to your goals?*

Think back to chemistry class again. Do you remember the diagram of a cell with the cell membrane, nucleus and cell wall? Well, that cell wall is the way nutrients like proteins and carbs are carried into the cell for consumption. A deficiency in fatty acids affects the permeability of the cell wall making it difficult for nutrients to move back and forth, interrupting your metabolism. Poor nutrient delivery = poor metabolism = poor results. It's extremely important to make sure the omega-3 you take is not only

manufactured properly to keep the integrity of the fat, but to make sure the ratio of DHA/EPA (which are types of omega and fatty acids) is most beneficial to you as well. Studies have shown that both substances have a positive effect on body functions.

3. VITAMIN D: It's not just for your bones! Vitamin D is insanely important for immune function and regulating all mineral absorption in the body. Between living inside and the widespread use of sunblock, most people don't get nearly enough sunlight to support natural production of Vitamin D in the body so a supplement is absolutely recommended. YOU CANNOT HAVE PROPER IMMUNE OR HORMONE FUNCTION WITHOUT IT. Make sure to get it in liquid form which is better and more effective for absorption than pills.

4. ADRENAL SUPPORT: As we know, the adrenal glands take on the burden of our everyday lives and chronic stress, causing them to constantly pump out adrenal hormones which can lead to adrenal fatigue and a host of other issues as we discussed earlier in this book. You must make sure you're doing everything possible to support and protect your adrenal glands as they can lead to ALL metabolic and health problems. Most people don't know this, but thyroid damage and conditions like hypothyroidism are actually *symptoms* of a hyperactive stress response from your adrenals. Obviously, it's impossible to avoid stress completely so the best thing we can do is to make sure we take the steps necessary to both mitigate stress and protect our adrenals. While a doctor can diagnose adrenal fatigue and make recommendations for treatment, I recommend everyone take an adrenal support formulation. If your adrenals aren't working properly, your fat loss potential is going to be severely hindered, if not rendered completely futile.

5. ESSENTIAL AMINO ACIDS: Among the nutritional problems most women face is not getting enough protein. Protein is not only the building block of muscle, it's the foundation of many metabolic processes and used to transport nutrients in and out of your cells. Protein deficiency = metabolic deficiency. This is not helpful when we are trying to build muscle, burn fat, and shape our bodies. Yes, I get it. You are busy and it's hard to stick to such a rigorous eating schedule. Trust me, I know firsthand the type of commitment it takes and understand sometimes life gets in the way. While I encourage you to eat whole foods several times a day, I also understand there are times when you just cannot do so. This is where this supplement comes in. Research shows any time you go beyond a four hour window without eating protein, you increase the chances of your metabolism becoming catabolic due to lack of certain amino acids such as leucine. What this means is your body starts to use protein for energy and begins tapping into protein stores which can have a massive effect on our lean muscle mass. As hard as it is to build muscle, the last thing we want to do is have it waste away, especially because muscle is our metabolic machine that burns fat and uses calories even when we're at rest. Eating a protein rich meal every few hours is ideal to avoid this happening. However, the most important part of this concept is getting in essential amino acids every few hours. Being prepared is key to your success. If you know you are going to miss meals, or even think there is a possibility you will, this type of supplement is your best friend.

Getting results the right way is not rocket science; it simply requires understanding our physiology and what the body needs to work right. Our bodies are incredible machines and operate remarkably well when we give them what they need. If you're serious about your goals and want to learn more on this topic, refer to the resources at the back of the book to request a customized supplement recommendation. I offer this free for anyone interested, not just my clients, because I know how dramatically the right supplements can impact people's lives. It has changed my life—which is why I am so passionate about sharing this knowledge. ★

Emily Frisella>>

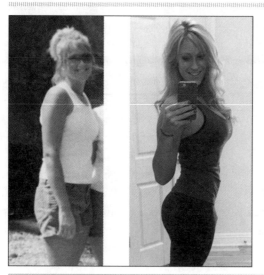

Emily Frisella, age 33

CEO/Creator, Fit Home & Health

Began working out at age 27

Favorite happy meal: Lasagna with garlic bread

"It's a lifestyle, not a 'diet.' It allows you to enjoy life while working towards your goals. When I work out I feel like a strong, powerful, badass bitch ready to take on life!"

Emily's Story: My name is Emily Frisella, Creator and CEO of Fit Home & Health. My mission is to help others become healthier by using real world recipes for busy lives by creating cookbooks with meals made simple. I began my journey to becoming more serious about my health seven years ago. I bought all sorts of healthy eating magazines and cookbooks to bring some fresh ideas into my kitchen instead of the standard chicken and broccoli most trainers promote.

Looking through these magazines and cookbooks led to nothing but total frustration because nearly all the recipes called for an insane amount of ingredients, items that were not easy to find, would cost an arm and a leg or took way too long to prepare. Like most women, I was busy with the career I had at the time, running a household, keeping a gym routine and had a wedding flower business on the side at the time. I was way too busy to spend two hours prepping a meal for dinner. I needed healthy, quick, and ingredient-friendly meals I could get in one trip to the grocery store. Then it happened. I was so frustrated at this fact I said, "Screw this, I'm writing my own damn recipes!" This is when Fit Home & Health was born. Two of my cookbooks will be released mid-2016 with additional books in 2017. These cookbooks are a blueprint to creating healthy recipes your whole family—even your kids—will enjoy. It's about a lifestyle, not a diet. You need recipes which work with your lifestyle, not make it more difficult.

Since I was tackling the obstacle of creating healthy meals I felt great but I knew I was still missing out on some key factors:

1) How to train properly for my goals

2) What to eat & how often to eat

3) Proper supplementation

I knew I wouldn't reach my goals just by eating one healthy meal at dinner each night. I knew I wasn't training as effectively as I could for optimal results. And I knew that I needed a more structured supplementation plan. I knew this from having been an athlete all my life, playing multiple sports from age five through college. I was always very active but had a poor diet which consisted of barely eating throughout the day then having one huge meal at dinner which was sometimes healthy, sometimes not. It didn't get me results then and wasn't getting me results now.

I was frustrated. I was training five days a week for two hours a day. I weighed 140 pounds at 5'11." I was very active, had a terrible diet, and used zero supplements. I was skinny fat. Period. I was ready for a change.

Fast forward to fall 2014. I became more serious than ever about my health. I had been working out for five or six years but I had different goals this time: I wanted to be fit and strong, not diet and exercise to be "skinny." I was tired of all the effort and getting no results. Therefore, I knew that I had to find a coach to help me. Not just 'a' coach. I needed 'the' coach. As we all know social media is at the forefront of society and one evening I was looking through 'fitness' hashtags and pages on Instagram and I came across this woman with the user name of @ BikiniBossTheresa; she was tall, blonde, lean, and had great content. I read through several of her posts and I could tell she wasn't the "industry standard."

She had children, a husband, and an active family life, ran her businesses, and had a true grasp on a busy woman's life. She spoke of consistency, balance, and how to incorporate fitness into your demanding life and I thought to myself, "Wait...what the?!?...Is this woman a normal person who actually gets it?!?" So many coaches I have seen in the past were all fitness and diet, 24/7 and never thought of balancing other things in life and were therefore rude and unforgiving of any 'hiccups' in your plan or adjustments that needed to be made. But I could tell Theresa got it. She understood life's challenges and obstacles and how to incorporate an effective fitness routine and manageable diet into your life to reach your goals. And that's exactly what I wanted.

I looked through more of her posts and saw some of the workouts she did and I honestly felt so pissed I hadn't found her sooner! Ha-ha. In the past I would kill myself doing cardio for forty-five minutes a day, lifting weights for an hour, five to six times a week and eating 900-1000 calories a day. So as you can imagine I was always hungry and physically ran down and guess what…I also lacked results! So frustrating!

I was ready to hire this woman and transform my cardio, skinny-fat body into a fitness body. I called her up the next day excited to talk with her but worried that since I was in Missouri and she was in Florida that it wouldn't be a match made in heaven. Theresa was so warm and receptive to my call. We chatted a bit and then she said those four magical words to me, "I do online training." YES!! The heavens opened, I heard angels singing, and also heard the fat on my body screaming in fear. We talked for a half hour or so which is covering a lot of ground if you've ever heard one of us talk. I couldn't decide which of us spoke faster. She shared my enthusiasm and excitement and understood everything I expressed—from joy to frustration—because she too had been there before. I signed up as soon as I hung up the phone. To say I was pumped is an understatement.

I received my nutrition and training plan shortly after signing up. The program looked awesome! Clean, crisp and easy to follow. The first email included a note from Theresa, my nutrition plan, training, and what truly was impressive is that she included videos of every exercise included in my training plan so there was no confusion. I printed out the spreadsheets and also took screen shots on my phone so I could easily access them during my workouts so I knew what was next.

Within the first week I felt better—mentally and physically. I was so excited to be taking these steps to make myself better. At the two-week mark I saw my body changing; inches were lost, my booty was popping, and I was smiling. I always struggled with my training. I knew how to lift but was left confused as to how many sets, reps, heavy weight, lightweight, and intensity. There were so many articles I read over the last decade and all of them would tell you something different.

The lifting and cardio Theresa assigned me were totally different. I would be in and out of the gym in about an hour. I did little to no cardio, ate a ton of nutritious food, and lifted weights according to my goals.

"Trust the process." You always hear that but that was hard for me to grasp based upon past experiences. It was different working with Theresa though. She was providing me the tools to reach my goals but she too had transformed herself. Clearly she knew what she was doing. So, for once, I finally trusted the process. Best Decision Ever! As I said earlier I was sitting at 140 lbs., 5'11", and skinny fat. Now I am sitting at 157 lbs. at 5'11". Let me repeat: I gained seventeen pounds, lost several inches, and the whole composition of my body changed. Getting in shape and simply losing weight are two totally different things. It took me trusting the process to realize that.

I learned that forty-five minutes of cardio five days a week was unnecessary and actually went against my goals. I was also often lifting too heavy for too long. I wasn't providing my body the proper nutrients and supplements. After more than a decade of yo-yo diets, conflicting weight training information, crazy amounts of cardio, and lack of use or timing of supplements everything was coming together.

I was empowered to take control of my body. I now had a "Bible to a Bikini Body" at my fingertips! The training, supplements, and nutrition were all aligned. I love that I have all these things, yet I still get a "Happy Meal" once a week which is key to keeping me on track and a coach who understands there is life outside the four walls of a gym and we all don't have hours every day to spend there.

Life is busy. Period. We all have our own type of crazy, chaotic, hectic schedules with career, family, kids, and events…it never ends. But this lifestyle I have now adopted is something that I love doing. I am spending less time in the gym and seeing greater results. It is not only helping me to reach my goals physically but also helps me perform better with my business and in my everyday life.

When you treat your body well, it returns the favor. ★

Emily Frisella
IG @EmilyFrisella
Fit Home & Health Creator/CEO. www.fithomeandhealth.com

Goal Weight = Sexy AF

PART

3

Before you start reading this section, I want you to stop what you are doing, close your eyes and imagine the body you have always wanted. Picture vividly the toned arms and shoulders, defined abs, nice round lifted butt, lean and sexy legs, nice smooth skin and a sexy sculpted back. Now imagine that body is yours because it will be. One of the first steps to getting a Bikini Boss body is accepting the fact that you can. Bikini models are not born with insanely fit bodies. However, they have learned the secrets to transform their bodies into aesthetic masterpieces, and you can, too. This section will teach you the most important and often overlooked secrets to transforming your body, no matter what your fitness level is, how many kids you've had, or how many programs you have tried in the past.

I will tell you though, from first-hand experience, you must have a positive mental attitude toward your body and your progress to get there. I've seen so many women make such great progress but they give up halfway there. Our bodies are amazing machines, and they are capable of some pretty incredible transformations, but they take some times. Cut yourself some slack and focus on the positive results you're getting and everything will come together in the end. You can't expect to start a program and wake up a week later with a bikini model's body. We've already covered all this in part two but you need to remind yourself of this daily until you get it.

To develop this type of physique, we have to recondition your metabolism, take your muscles through specific growth and recovery phases, and give your body time to adapt to your new program and lifestyle. And yes, I said lifestyle. THIS IS NOT A DIET! All of the tips, secrets, and strategies I will give you in the following chapters will work, but you cannot expect to maintain an incredible physique if you completely fall off the wagon and go back to your old, unhealthy, and undesirable habits. If you're like me, this won't be an issue because once you feel great and look incredible, you won't ever want to go back. Now let's get to the good stuff!

The Program > > >

CHAPTER 9

Lift More than Your Groceries

EVERYTHING WE'VE LAID out so far has simply been to get your mind ready for the good stuff—the PROGRAM! And I'm going to start by talking about one of the most important factors in transforming your body: THE WORKOUT. Now, I know many of you will be starting at different fitness levels and different levels of conditioning, but regardless of the starting point, the goal is to get you to the same finish line; and trust me, we will! I am going to use a variety of terms in the next few chapters, and it will make your life a lot easier if I just define them now. You can refer back to this section as needed.

- **REPETITION (REP)**—the number of times you complete a specific exercise. i.e.: 12 curls= 12 reps
- **SET**—a group of repetitions you complete continuously. It can be just one exercise or a group of different exercises, i.e.: 12 curls, 12 squats, 12 rows = 1 set
- **REP RANGE**—the number of reps you should aim for during a specific set, i.e.: 10-12 reps
- **WEIGHT RANGE**—the range of weight you should be using for a specific exercise
- **SUPER SET**—a technique where you perform two exercises in a row with next to no rest in between.
- **MOVEMENT PREP**—warm up exercises used to get your muscles and nervous system ready for the workout. Typically done with little or no weight, i.e.: walking lunges, push-ups, planks, air squats, etc.
- **EPOC (EXCESS POST-OXYGEN**

CONSUMPTION)—the metabolic state your body is in after a super high-intensity exercise which creates such an oxygen debt that your body takes up to 36 hours to fully recover. EPOC is ideal for optimal fat loss physiology.

- **GLYCOGEN –** A chain of carbohydrate (sugar) molecules stored within the muscle cell. It is the main fuel for muscles when working hard. Basically, anything you do in the gym is fueled by glycogen.

- **INTRAMUSCULAR TRIGLYCERIDES** – This is the fat which lives inside of the muscle. When most of us think of fat, we are thinking of subcutaneous fat—the kind you can pinch. Intramuscular fat is more like the marbling on a steak. Intramuscular triglycerides are the main fuel used by muscles that will be active for long periods of time such as a six-hour hike.

First, I need you to understand something very important; you will never have a bikini model's body without the right kind of workout. This bears repeating: *You will NEVER have a bikini model's body without the right kind of workout.* Far too many women think they can get the body they want by doing tons of cardio and lifting tiny pink weights. This kind of training (mixed with the right nutrition strategy) can help you lose some fat, but it will NEVER put

enough stress on your body to build muscle or truly change your physique. If you only want to lose scale weight and look "skinny fat," then keep doing hours of endless cardio and lifting the tiny pink weights in Zumba class. But if you really want that bikini model body, you will be lifting HEAVY weights at some point in your program so you need to get it through your head right now. At this point, I know some of you are thinking:

> *"But Theresa, won't lifting heavy weights make me bulky? I don't want to look like one of those female bodybuilders. I still want to look feminine…"*

I understand your concern and I used to train using super light weights and dozens of reps. But, as I've already discussed, the reality is it wasn't until I found a coach who had me lifting some VERY heavy weights that my body really started to change in the ways I wanted it to. The reason has to do with the physiology of how muscles REALLY change. A muscle is made up of about 75 to 80 percent water, 15 to 20 percent protein, and the rest comes from about 1 percent each of carbohydrates, fats, and inorganic molecules. The most variable components are the fat and water content, as the more fat you're carrying, the less water there is. Just think of how much smaller a lean chicken breast gets when you cook it compared to a fatty steak. This is why good hydration is one of the most important things you can do to keep your muscles looking sexy. So step one to building more muscle is as simple as drinking more water.

When it comes to what you do in the gym, there are really only TWO main stressors that make muscles grow—high muscular tension and high metabolic buildup. Let me explain these activities.

1. HIGH TENSION (HEAVY WEIGHT)— The main stress to build the 15 to 20 percent of our muscles that is actually protein is high tension. That means lifting weights that you can only lift five times or less. If you can lift the weight more, you aren't truly maximizing the building of muscle protein.

2. HIGH METABOLIC BUILDUP (HIGH REPS)— This is what happens when you "feel the burn" during a workout, usually after 30 to 45 seconds of continuous tension. This is related to the glycogen component to muscles—which is only 1 percent of the size of a muscle.

It makes a lot more sense to base our training on getting 20 percent of our muscle to grow compared to only 1 percent. This is why lifting heavy is so important—it targets the muscular components that grow the most. Now some of you who aren't new to training may have heard of using moderate rep ranges (8 to 12 reps). This is a good happy medium to get both the "heavy weights" and the "feel the burn"

adaptations. But what you'll see is we use a variety of rep ranges to really maximize all of the muscular adaptations possible.

1 THE WORKOUT: IGNITE, SCULPT, SHRED!

The Boss to Bikini workout is a ninety-day program designed to radically change your body and teach you how to work out like a bikini model. It is broken down into three phases, each one lasting thirty days.

IGNITE

This phase is a general conditioning program designed to get you working out more frequently, and getting you accustomed to lifting heavier weights than you've used in the past. Coupled with our fat loss nutrition programs, this phase will boost your metabolism so you should see the inches start to drop quickly, while simultaneously building your strength and endurance. You will be in the gym five days a week during the Ignite phase. Since it's a cardiovascular demanding workout you will not need to do any additional cardio in phase one.

Your rep range will be a little higher during this phase compared to the other stages of the program. The main focus of the workouts should be increasing balance, core stabilization and all-over muscular stability. This is the most important phase because it preps the nervous system and muscular system for the more intense and physically demanding workouts in the next phase and helps to prevent injury. You can't build anything substantial without a good foundation! Learning proper form and execution of the exercises during this period is crucial to your future success.

SCULPT

This is the phase that really sets the Boss to Bikini program apart from the others available today. In the Sculpt phase we are going to switch up the diet and put you into lean muscle building mode. You'll also see the weights get heavier in the gym. This is not only the best way to build muscle but provides a nice side benefit by giving you confidence from doing something you didn't realize you were capable of doing. Many of our clients LOVE the feeling they get when then walk into a gym and are lifting weights heavier than guys twice their size.

You should now be using a heavy enough weight that you cannot complete more than four to eight reps without being forced to take an adequate rest between sets. A weight range of 15 to 40 pounds is a good guide line to start; however, don't be surprised if you end up using somewhere between 50 to 100-pound weights for your leg exercises after your first two weeks! You should start off lower and increase as the weeks progress. I want to stress that you should be lifting a weight where you can barely finish no more than 4 to 8 reps while still keeping good form.

You need to push yourself in this phase to go as heavy as possible or you will not get the best results. I always suggest you print out your workouts and bring the list to a gym so you can track the weight you're lifting. Even though you'll be doing the same workout for four weeks in a row, you always want to keep progressing by increasing weight so tracking it gives you a good goal for each subsequent week.

Some of you may be able to lift heavier than the weight range I have listed. As long as you are keeping good form, that's great!! Go as high as you need to bring the muscles to fatigue during your set. For example, when I first started lifting heavy I started immediately with 35-pound squats (70 pounds total) and 100-pound deadlifts. Now I am up to more than 250 pounds on my deadlift! I was in pretty good shape before, so my body was ready to handle it. Not everyone will be in this condition until they have been lifting for a few weeks or maybe even months. Just make sure you use proper form, and don't overdo it—I cannot stress this enough! Injuries are not fun!

SHRED

After spending the last month building new lean muscle, now it's time to reveal it! Here we will switch you back to a fat-burning program, but you will have the added benefit of carrying extra muscle while doing so. The result will be a dramatically different body from the one you had when you started this program.

While I understand most of you will be working out with the ultimate goal of shedding unwanted body fat, you must first take your body through the proper muscular adaptation phases to ensure the muscles are ready for the type of exercise in this phase. Get ready to see all of your hard work come to fruition!

In this final phase, you will now start incorporating super high-intensity workouts into your routine to put your body into a state of metabolic shock known as EPOC (excess post oxygen consumption). This type of exercise will keep your body recovering from the workout and burning fat for up to 36 hours after you are done, even while you sleep!

We accomplish this by:

- Switching from heavy to a light-moderately heavy weight range
- Increasing the tempo (the time between reps) at which you perform the exercises…think speed
- Adding plyometric, "jump training," and high-intensity bursts throughout the workout
- Burning out the muscles and taking them to complete fatigue
- Switching from longer workouts to a high-intensity,–short-duration

workout, meaning if you are working out correctly, you should not be able to do more than 30 minutes of this type of intense exercise
- Introducing high-intensity interval training

An important thing to note is that this is EXACTLY how I train clients who are in competition. Everyone starts at a different place, but they all go through pretty much the same process once they desire to step on stage. The ones who have been with us for a long time and have competed in multiple body building events simply trade-off between different Sculpt and Shred phases we provide, depending on their weaknesses and their goals.

In the first two phases of the program, you will be increasing the weight load and decreasing the number of reps you complete as you progress. Finally, once you have moved successfully through the appropriate adaptation phases, <u>and you have the muscle to support it</u>, the LAST AND FINAL step is to switch to a super high-intensity fat-blasting workout.

> Everyone will progress differently on this program depending on their previous training frequency, intensity, and neuromuscular response. I know you want to have your dream
>
> *continued*

body RIGHT NOW but you need to remember making any significant progress with building muscle and burning fat takes a little time. That's why fitness models and athletes start training months before an actual show or event. I prefer to have AT LEAST six months of prep time with a woman before sending her out for her first competition. This is not a quick fix so I want you to stop and accept the fact that it will take a little time to sculpt your body. The great thing is—it will be totally worth it!! The way you will be training your body to become a machine will make it SO easy to keep your results instead of having to yo-yo diet all the time.

BEFORE YOU BEGIN!

It is so important for you to ALWAYS maintain proper form during your workouts. This is not only to make sure your muscles are firing correctly but also so you avoid serious injuries; especially when you are lifting heavy weight! Here are the most important tips to good form during workouts:

1. Always engage your core... ALWAYS! Pretend someone is going to punch you in the stomach. That's how I want you to keep your core during ALL exercises.

2. Shoulders open and chest out. You should not have your shoulders hunched and chest caved in... stick out those boobs!

3. Squeeze your glutes during every exercise, every single time! Not only is this better for your core stability, it will help to tighten up those butt muscles too! If you are doing leg or booty exercises and not squeezing your butt the entire time, it will not be as effective and you will be more vulnerable to back injury. If you have to, lower your weight and go nice and slow. Form is the most important factor in results.

4. BREATHE. Yes, this seems simple but many people hold their breath during exercise. This is not a good thing for many reasons. I tell my clients to stand in front of a mirror so they can watch themselves as they work out. You should feel air expand not just your ribcage, but down into your belly

5. In any squatting, lunging or bending exercises, don't let your knees collapse inwards. Make sure they stay lined up with the middle of the foot. Your knees should track right through your middle toe.

64

****AVOID THIS MISTAKE****

Do not over-train by adding a bunch of extra workouts and working out six to seven days per week! Over-training will ultimately defeat what you are trying to accomplish by adding too much physiological stress to your body and breaking down your muscles. It will actually lessen your fat burning hormones. Your body needs time to rest and recover. Muscles don't get bigger in the gym; they get bigger when you're recovering. And if you never get a chance to recover, your muscles NEVER GET A CHANCE TO GROW. More doesn't always equal better. If you currently have a sport or activity that you participate in, you don't want to do any more than one or two extra workouts a week on top of what you're already doing in our program.

A FEW MORE TIPS:

- Rest, don't nap between sets or when needed
- Drink plenty of water
- Take the recommended supplements
- Get a workout partner for more motivation and better results
- Lastly, have fun!

Why is movement so important? Lessons from the deep seas.

I'm going to ask you a question. Why do you need a brain? If you're like most people, you're going to give the obvious answer: to think. But believe it or not, this is completely wrong. The fundamental purpose of our brain and nervous system is to create complex and varied movement. About 90% of the brain's energy is used to keep us oriented in gravity. Only 10% is delegated to thinking, metabolism, and everything else. We can create computers that can out-think chess grandmasters, but we are still worlds away from creating computers that could move a chess piece with the dexterity of a six-month old child.

To really show how linked movement is to brain function, let's go underwater. There is a very primitive sea animal called a Sea Squirt. When it is born, the tadpole shaped organism has a very basic nervous system (only about 300 cells). At the start of its life, it swims along the ocean floor, looking for a suitable source of food and nutrients. Once it finds this, it plants its roots into the ground. It's next order of business? IT EATS AND DIGESTS ITS OWN BRAIN. Literally. Once it doesn't need to move anymore, it doesn't really need a brain anymore.

We obviously aren't primitive sea creatures, but our nervous systems aren't that different. There are numerous studies that have shown that EVERY part of the brain

works better with regular exercise. Yes, we are working out to look sexy AF, but don't be surprised if your day-to-day life finds better memory, concentration, focus, and cognitive performance. Exercise and quality movement has much further reaching benefits than we realize.

GETTING THE BODY READY—MOVEMENT PREP IS THE NEW WARM-UP

If you're anything like me, when you think of a "warm-up," you think back to your grade school and high school phys ed classes. You would jog a lap or two around the gym, hold a few stretches for about ten seconds, and then go right into whatever activity was scheduled for the day. The problem is none of this adequately gets the body ready for exercise. A warm-up is designed to help prepare your body for your workout, to maximize the benefits of the

workout, and almost more importantly, to prevent injury. Just as losing fat and building muscle takes time, healing damaged tissues takes time. If you strain a muscle it takes three months MINIMUM for that tissue to return back to 100 percent. And that's if you do everything right! There's no easier way to derail your progress than having to take a few weeks or months off of training.

The research shows that you want your warm-up to increase your body temperature, and to move your body through whatever ranges of motion you're going to be using in your workout. We recommend starting with five to ten minutes of continuous activity on a treadmill, elliptical, etc., just until you feel a light sweat and a mild increase in breathing rate. From here, I'll go into some full body dynamic movements to help take the joints through their full ranges of motion. The dynamic warm-up shouldn't take much more than five minutes. Some sample dynamic warm-up exercises are as follows:

66

■ PUSHUPS ■
5-10 slow and controlled reps

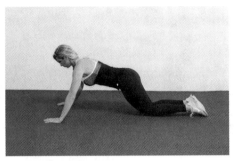

Pushup Start (Basic)

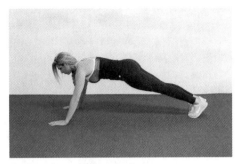

Pushup Start (Advanced)

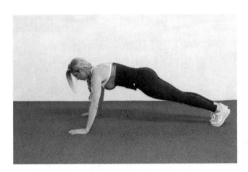

Pushup (Good alignment)

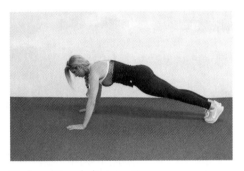

Pushup (Good alignment)

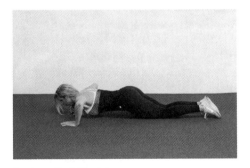

Pushup End (Basic)

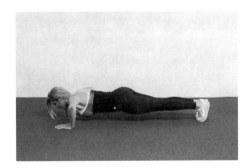

Pushup End (Advanced)

LIFT MORE THAN YOUR GROCERIES

WALKING LUNGES

10 reps per leg

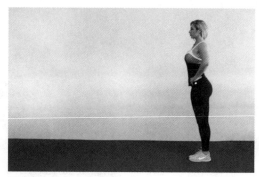

Walking Lunge (Start)

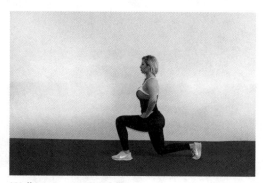

Walking Lunge (Middle)

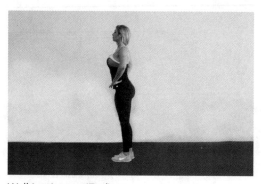

Walking Lunge (End)

■ BENCH DIPS ■
10 reps

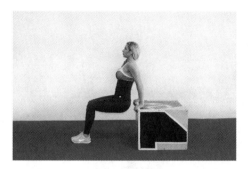

Bench Dip Start (Basic)

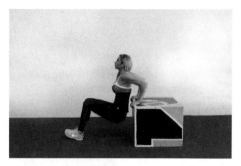

Bench Dip End (Basic)

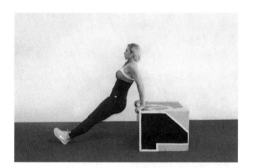

Bench Dip Start (Advanced)

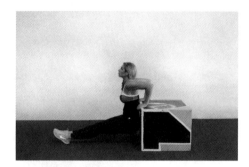

Bench Dip End (Advanced)

■ AIR SQUATS ■
20 reps

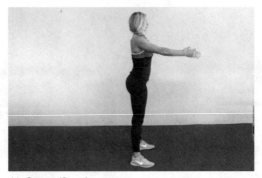

Air Squat (Start)

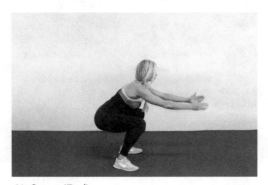

Air Squat (End)

70

◼ ARM SWINGS ◼

10 reps per arm, per direction

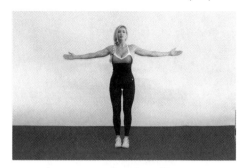

Arm Swings Cross Body (Start)

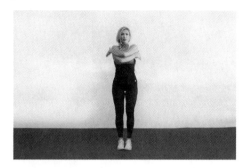

Arm Swings Cross Body (End)

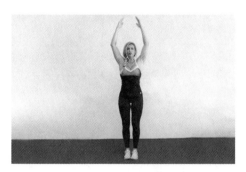

Arm Swings Overhead (Start)

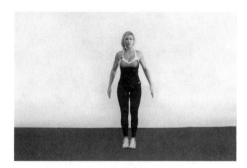

Arm Swings Overhead (End)

LIFT MORE THAN YOUR GROCERIES

◼ LEG SWINGS ◼
10 swings per leg

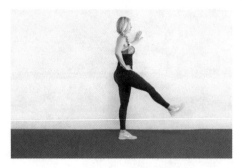

Leg Swings Back & Forth (Start)

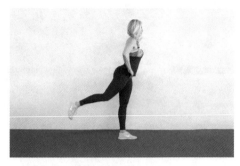

Leg Swings Back & Forth (End)

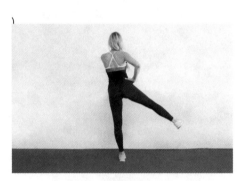

Leg Swings Cross Body (Start)

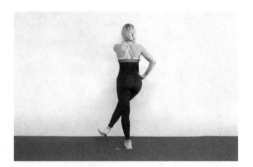

Leg Swings Cross Body (End)

▪ TOE KICKS ▪
10 kicks per leg

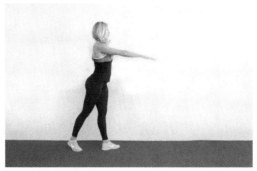

Toe Kicks (Start)

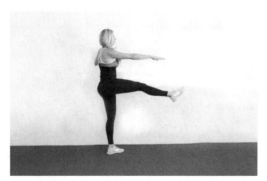

Toe Kicks (End)

LIFT MORE THAN YOUR GROCERIES

SHOULDER "DISLOCATES"

10 reps per hand position

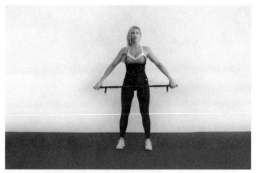

Shoulder "Dislocates" (Start)

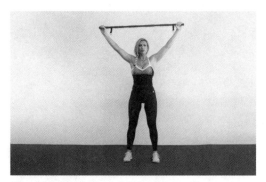

Shoulder "Dislocates" (Middle)

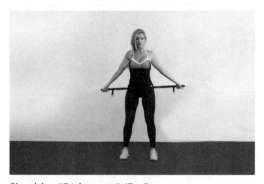

Shoulder "Dislocates" (End)

▪ KNEE-TO-CHEST ▪
10 reps per leg

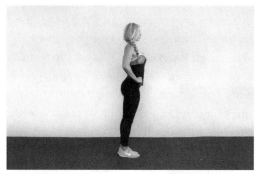

Knee-to-chest (Start)

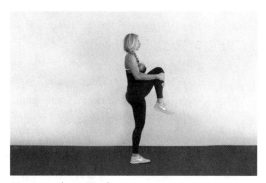

Knee-to-chest (End)

LIFT MORE THAN YOUR GROCERIES

THE NEW RULES OF STRETCHING

Almost everyone you see at the beginning of a workout, will be stretching to some degree. But believe it or not, study after study shows that this does more harm than good. Stretching relaxes muscles which is great if you're after relaxation, but not so good if you're trying to generate force. Actually, maximal strength is significantly decreased after prolonged stretching. Basically, stretching "turns down" how quickly and efficiently your nerves talk to your muscles. That's a good thing for increasing flexibility, but not effective for a complex workout. Actually, it increases the risk of injury. Yes, PROLONGED STATIC STRETCHING BEFORE YOUR WORKOUT INCREASES YOUR RISK OF INJURY. I'd rather not go out of my way to do anything that INCREASES injury.

On the other hand, your chances of injury are increased if your muscles are out of balance. So if something is too tight, we DO want to stretch it. In women, the most common tight muscles are usually the hip flexors, quads, and calves. (This is a by-product of wearing heels.) If you DO want to stretch something, pay attention to these commonly tight areas, and ONLY do static stretching after your workout, or on non-training days. Warmed up muscles do in fact stretch better, so I recommend stretching post workout.

And guess what? That ten to thirty second stretch you've been doing isn't cutting it. If you feel like you've been stretching the same tight muscle groups for years without making any progress, that's because the research shows it takes more than TWO MINUTES of continuous tension in a stretched position to get the muscles and tendons to change at the cellular level. I recommend picking the two or three muscle groups in your body that are the tightest, and dedicating the end of your workout to making them move better. Your body will thank you.

BUT SERIOUSLY THOUGH, WHERE'S THE CARDIO?

I'm sure most of you LOVE cardio but we need to talk about the different types and how they can affect you and your fitness and fat-loss goals. The first and most important thing to understand is that our bodies and metabolisms are not designed for long periods of VERY INTENSE steady state activity. Our genes evolved with two speeds: "All-day slow" (think walking and foraging) and "Fight-or-flight fast." We are good at going very hard for a short period, and very easy for long periods. But our physiology just doesn't like fairly hard for fairly long durations. There is actually emerging evidence showing high intensity marathon training having NEGATIVE inflammatory effects on cardiovascular health.

Endurance cardio (for our purposes, more than thirty minutes) where you go as hard as you can for as long as you can not only wears away at your muscle, but it can also cause a huge stress response in the body—which you should know by now is not a good thing! It's an old myth that you need to work out in the "cardio zone" to burn fat. This mind-set was perpetuated by the calorie counting method of weight loss (old paradigm); if you burn more than you consume you will be "skinny." However, as most of you know, the only thing this mindset accomplishes is making you skinny FAT. If you want to get a bikini model's body your goal should be fat loss, not weight loss. Endurance cardio is good for losing weight because you lose weight—including fat, water, and muscle. That is not our goal. You cannot afford to lose muscle! So, you decide:

Weight loss = soft and puffy vs. Fat loss = sculpted and sexy

You're probably wondering then, what do I do for cardio?

There is a disconnect between what we THINK we need to do to keep our heart healthy, and what is actually necessary to keep our heart healthy. If your heart rate is elevated for an adequate amount of time (not too much, not too little), you get cardiovascular benefits. Here's the secret though: you can get your heart rate up just as easily (usually more easily) by strength training, than you can by using steady-state cardio. If your friends, family, or even doctor tell you that you HAVE to do traditional cardio for heart health, they're sadly mistaken.

I know some of you really enjoy things like biking, swimming, spin class, etc. so I will explain how to use cardio properly to your advantage.

BURN FAT FOR AN HOUR? OR A COUPLE OF DAYS?

Here's where the magic of the Boss to Bikini program comes in. You can burn fat while you sleep. When your metabolism is elevated, you're using more energy. That means burning more calories. And guess what? Some exercises raise your metabolism more than others. When you perform steady state cardio, your heart rate and metabolism will recover shortly after the workout. When you perform high intensity interval (HIIT) training, your metabolism stays elevated for HOURS after your workout. And when you perform metabolic resistance training (the type found in our Ignite and Shred programs), your metabolism stays elevated for DAYS. You heard me right, days. That means if I do the right kind of workout on Monday, I'm still burning extra fat from it on Wednesday. If I had my choice, I'd focus my efforts on the workouts that give the most bang for my buck. And I do.

HIIT cardio- (High Intensity Interval Training) – This is the only cardio I do and what I prefer my clients do. That's because it is the type of exercise our bodies were designed for—high intensity bursts of energy followed by adequate rest and recovery periods. So what exactly does HIIT mean? SPRINTS! That doesn't necessarily mean running, but it does mean FULL OUT EFFORT of any continuous activity (including running, biking, StairMaster, etc.) for somewhere between fifteen and sixty seconds followed by a rest period of at least the same amount of time, if not more. And when I say rest, I mean taking it down to almost no exertion level. For example, I will set the treadmill on 11.5 speed and do a sprint for thirty seconds. Then, I jump off, standing on the sides, for a thirty- to forty-five-second rest. I usually do a few sets of these mixed in with some brisk walking.

A few tips on sprinting: If you are new to working out and have not been running, DO NOT START WITH SPRINTING. Fast running can put forces through your legs in excess of four to five times your body weight! If you try this and your body can't handle it, you WILL get injured. The reason you see so many injuries in runners is because they do more than the body is prepared to handle. Running per se isn't bad for your joints, but it is bad for joints that haven't been properly prepared.

If your body CAN handle the forces or running, start by doing one or two 10-second sprints and build up… and you don't have to be on an 11.5 pace on the treadmill. Set it at a number that is as fast as YOU can safely run and increase it and the time as you feel more conditioned. You should really push yourself though. Just running fast is not sprinting and will not have the same hormonal effect on fat loss.

NOW, I'M GOING TO TOTALLY CONTRADICT MYSELF….

I recommend you do slow, casual, leisurely walking every week.

"But Theresa, you just told me this kind of exercise is almost useless for fat loss…"

And it is. But that's not why you're doing it. Depending on which study you look at, hunter-gatherers (think, YOUR genes), were on their feet, walking anywhere from twelve to sixteen miles PER DAY, outside, barefoot or in some very minimalistic foot covering. Our genes are designed for us to be on our feet, and moving. Our walking recommendation isn't so much about your burning more fat, but it is related to stress relief, hormonal balance, getting some sun exposure, and just moving in a very natural, human way.

Studies have also showed that the metabolic "sweet spot" (think of the speed on your car where you get the best MPG) is just under three mph. That's not very fast. Again, speed, raising the heart rate, and burning calories is NOT the goal. Go for a casual walk with the dog. Or take your kids to the park. Or go for a walk with your significant other. Stop and smell the roses. A healthy mind is integral to a healthy body, and walking is a way to hack into this innate form of relaxation. On one of your days off, the Boss to Bikini plan involves one sixty-minute CASUAL walk every week. ★

Bikini Boss
BOOTY SECRETS

Before introducing the program, I want to share a few secrets to getting a great butt. Have you ever looked at bikini models and wondered how they got their butts so perfect? Nice and round, lifted, shapely and NO cellulite? Don't feel bad, I used to, too! If you know any of them or follow them on social media you will learn that many of them didn't always look that way. The reason they all have perfect butts is because they have learned how to work out to transform their glutes into the perfect bikini booty.

I myself have gone through this transformation. In fact, this was one of the hardest areas for me to see change; until I learned the Secrets to achieving this but now I'm pleased to say I have a booty of envy! Here are the most important tips.

Stretch your hip flexors. Most of us have tight hip flexors from sitting at work, school, while driving, etc. Hip flexors are the primary mover that is the antagonist (opposite action) to your glutes. If they are extremely tight, they will keep your glutes from turning on properly during exercise, rendering your workouts pretty much pointless. Always stretch your hips and hip flexors right before and after any leg/booty workouts.

Use your glutes, NOT your back. A lot of girls end up hyperextending their backs when doing glute exercises. This creates two simultaneous problems: it under-stimulates the glutes and overstresses the lower back. Brace your abs and keep your lower back rock solid when doing your glute exercises.

Squeeze your glutes all the time!!! I cannot stress how much this helps. Just as when your hip flexors are tight they inhibit the glutes, conversely, if you don't tighten your glutes you won't lengthen your hip flexors or ever correct the issue. When I say all the time, I mean it! Squeeze them when you're standing at work, at the store, sitting in the car, and ALWAYS during workouts, especially butt and leg workouts. I'm serious, the more you work the glute muscles, the better they will look.

LIFT MORE THAN YOUR GROCERIES

Glutes are responsible for two entirely different movements. I'm sure you've heard of the gluteus maximus (or "glute max"). This is the muscle that makes up the majority of what we think of when we think of the glutes. Its main job is to kick the leg back, and a little to the side. Think of a movement like skating. But the gluteus medius (or "glute med") sits on the side of the hip, and is responsible for kicking your leg straight out to the side. Think of a side-shuffle or abduction. You need to train BOTH of them to get that bikini model booty. Think of the glute med as what makes your booty round, and the glute max as what makes it perky.

You can work out glutes almost every day. There has been this myth going around the fitness industry for years that you can only work out your muscle groups once per week. FALSE! You will be shocked at how much faster they respond when they get used more frequently. Some muscle groups have different combinations of muscle fibers that allow them to not fatigue as easily. No one would ever say to only use your tongue or eye muscles once a week, but we seem to think our other muscles need absurd amounts of rest. I personally work my glutes three to four times a week.

Boss to Bikini

90-DAY WORKOUT PROGRAM

PHASE 1: IGNITE

DAYS ONE AND FOUR			DAYS TWO AND FIVE			DAY THREE		
Exercise Name	Sets	Time per set	Exercise Name	Sets	Time per set	Exercise Name	Sets	Time per set
Plank	4	1 min	Pushups (Knees are fine)	4	1 min	Walking Abduction w/ Band	4	1 min
Walking Lunges	4	1 min	Bicep Curls (Bands)	4	1 min	Sumo Squats w/ Dumbbells	4	1 min
Glute Bridge w/ Pulse	4	1 min	Tricep Kickbacks (Bands)	4	1 min	Calf Raises	4	1 min
Squat Jacks	4	1 min	Alt. DB Shoulder Press	4	1 min	Side Plank (30 sec per side)	4	1 min
Air Squats	4	1 min	Plank Shoulder Touch	4	1 min	Bicycle Kicks	4	1 min
Band Rows	4	1 min	Jumping Jacks	4	1 min	Physio Ball Hamstring Curl	4	1 min
Toe Reach	4	1 min	Physio Ball Pass	4	1 min	Glute Kickbacks w/ Ankle Weights	4	1 min

DAY ONE			DAY TWO			DAY THREE			DAY FOUR		
Exercise Name	Sets	Reps	Exercise Name	Sets	Reps	Exercise Name	Sets	Reps	Exercise Name	Sets	Reps
A1) Sumo Deadlift	5	5	A1) Narrow Pushup (10 sec negative)	4	6	Barbell Squat	4	8	Pushups	4	Failure
A2) Tuck Jumps	5	30s	A2) Dumbell Bent over Row	4	6	DumbBell Lunge	4	8	Seated Row (neutral grip)	4	15
B1) Leg Press	5	5	B1) Barebell Shoulder Press	4	6	Leg Extension (single leg)	4	10	Dumbell Shoulder Press	4	12
B2) Lunge Jumps	4	30s	B2) Wide Grip Lat pulldown	4	6	Hamstring curl (single leg)	4	10	Pronated grip lat pulldown	4	12
C1) Leg Extension	4	10	C1) Lateral Shoulder Raise	4	15	Seated Abduction	4	15	Front Shoulder Raise	4	15
C2) Leg Curl	4	10	C2) Tricep Press downs	4	12	Calf Raise (Standing, heels touching)	4	20	Tricep Overhead Press	4	12
D1) "Fire Hydrants"	3	15	D1) Single Leg glute Bridge	4	15 (per leg)	A1) Side-lying "clamshell"	3	15	A1) Glute Bridge w/ band abduction	3	15
D2) Banana Rocks	3	30	D2) Reverse Crunch (Arms on chest)	4	30	A2) Banana Hold	3	30s	A2) Hanging Leg raise	3	15

LIFT MORE THAN YOUR GROCERIES

	DAY ONE			DAY TWO			DAY THREE			DAY FOUR			DAY FIVE		
Exercise Name	Sets	Reps	Exercise Name	Sets	Reps	Exercise Name	Sets	Reps	Exercise Name	Sets	Reps	Exercise Name	Sets	Reps
A1) Jumping Jacks	3	20	Pushups	2	20	"Kickstand" Jumps	2	20	Close grip pushup	3	20	Walking lunges	2	30
A2) Hip Swings	3	20	Side Shuffle	2	1 min	"Up & Down" Planks	2	20	Plie Air Squats	3	20	Squat Abduction side kick	2	10 (per leg)
A3) Air Squats	3	20	Plank "Hitchiker"	2	1 min	Toe Kicks	2	20	Explosive Bosu pushup	5	20	Single leg deadlift (wt. in opp. Hand)	4	12
Walking Lunges	5	10 (per leg)	Decline PB push up	4	15	Speed hammer curl (fr. Squat)	5	20	Skull crushers	5	10	Kettlebell swing	4	12
Plie Squats (weighted)	5	20	Static Squat w/ rear delt fly	4	10	Rope curls	5	10	Wide grip lat pulldown	5	10	DB bent over row	4	6
Box Jumps	5	20	Lateral raise w/ pause	4	8	Seated calf raise	5	12	Cable tri pulldown	5	12	Hanging leg lifts	4	30

BOSS TO BIKINI

Continued on next page

DAY ONE			DAY TWO			DAY THREE			DAY FOUR			DAY FIVE		
Hip Thrusts	5	10	Banana Rocks	4	30	Standing Calf raise	5	30	Plank w/ alt. tri kickback	5	10 (per arm)	"Curtsey" step up (bench)	4	15 (per leg)
Squat Jacks (w/ Med ball)	5	30	DB Push through	4	10	Reverse grip pullup (assisted if needed)	5	5	Bulgarian split squat jumps	5	10 (per leg)	Hamstring curls	4	10
V-Ups (Weighted)	5	50	Sit up w/ reach	4	15	Preacher curl	5	8				Stiff-legged deadlifts	4	30
			Plank Shoulder touch	4	50	Reverse plank rollout PB	5	15				Abduction machine hover	4	30
			Push Press	4	8	Cable glute kickbacks	5	20 (per leg)						
HIIT Intervals		20 mins				HIIT Intervals		20 mins				HIIT Intervals		20 mins

LIFT MORE THAN YOUR GROCERIES

*NOTE ON HIIT (HIGH-INTENSITY INTER-VAL TRAINING). We are going to give you some options as to how you do your HIIT sessions. After your workouts on days 1, 3 and 5, you are going to do a twenty-minute interval session. Most commonly, I'll have girls do these with treadmill sprints, the stepper, the spin bike or the rowing machine. But if your gym has access to more equipment, go ahead and get creative! We've had girls do their HIIT intervals with sprints on actual running tracks or stairs, use battle ropes, weighted sleds, kettlebells swings, and more! Here are some sample HIIT templates that you can use:

HIIT 20A – 15 seconds hard, 45 seconds easy (15 rounds)

HIIT 20B – 30 seconds hard, 30 seconds easy (15 rounds)

HIIT 20C – 60 seconds hard, 2 minutes easy (5 rounds)

HIIT 20D – 90 seconds hard, 90 seconds easy (5 rounds)

HIIT 20E – 2 minutes hard, 1 minute easy (5 rounds)

(All HIIT sessions have a 2.5 minute warm up and cooldown)

SPECIAL BONUS: My Favorite Booty Builders. In addition to the comprehensive 90-day workout plan, I've decided to share some of my favorite booty building exercises with you. When working with my clients in competition, I will usually add some extra exercises for weak areas that need a little extra help. Since I don't get to see you in person like I do with my competition clients, I can't know what your "weakest" area is. So I'm going to assume your booty could use a little extra help—this is the case for most of us! Even though I've designed this 90-day program to be comprehensive, and you will get amazing results just doing the plan exactly as is, if you're the kind of person who will do a little extra regardless, let me steer you in the right direction.

BONUS BOOTY BUILDERS. Choose two "Transverse glute strength" exercises and two "Lateral glute strength" exercises (four exercises total). Alternate back and forth between a "transverse" exercise and a "lateral" exercise, and repeat the four-exercise cycle, three times at the end of every workout. (Do three circuits of the four exercises.)

TRANSVERSE GLUTE STRENGTH
▪ GLUTE BRIDGES ▪
30 reps

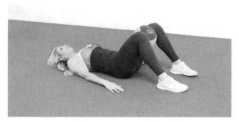

Glute Bridge with Adduction (Start)

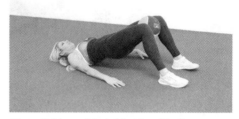

Glute Bridge with Adduction (End)

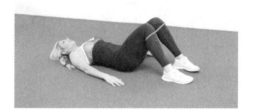

Glute Bridge with Abduction (Start)

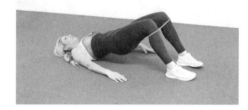

Glute Bridge with Abduction (End)

LIFT MORE THAN YOUR GROCERIES

◾ ELEVATED GLUTE BRIDGES ◾
30 reps

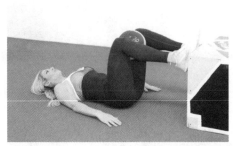

Elevated Glute Bridge with Adduction (Start)

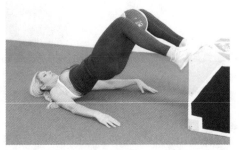

Elevated Glute Bridge with Adduction (End)

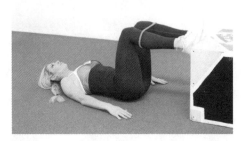

Elevated Glute Bridge with Abduction (Start)

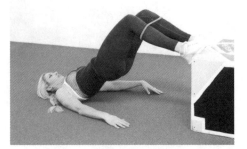

Elevated Glute Bridge with Adduction (End)

HIP THRUSTS

30 reps

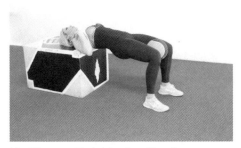

Hip Thrust with Adduction (Start)

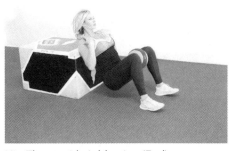

Hip Thrust with Adduction (End)

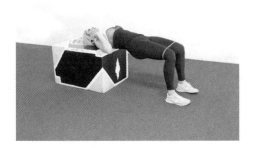

Hip Thrust with Abduction (Start)

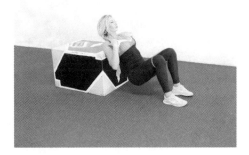

Hip Thrust with Abduction (End)

LIFT MORE THAN YOUR GROCERIES

■ FLOOR BRIDGES ■
15 reps per side

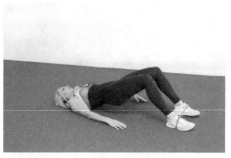

Floor Bridge with Single Leg Hip Flexion
(Start)

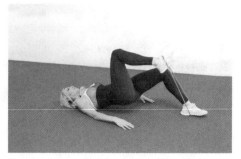

Floor Bridge with Single Leg Hip Flexion
(End)

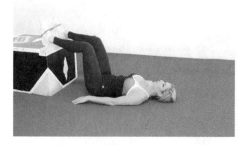

Elevated Bridge with Single Leg Hip Flexion
(Start)

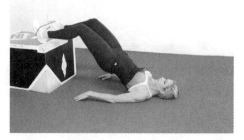

Elevated Bridge with Single Leg Hip Flexion
(Middle)

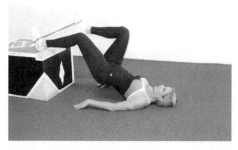

Elevated Bridge with Single Leg Hip Flexion
(End)

90

STATIC HIP TRUSTS

15 reps per side

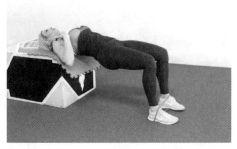

Static Hip Thrust with Single Hip Flexion
(Start)

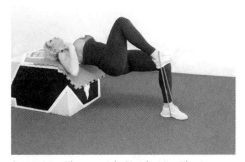

Static Hip Thrust with Single Hip Flexion
(End)

■ STATIC ELEVATED BRIDGE ■

15 reps per side

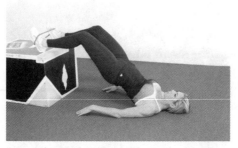

Static Elevated Bridge with Single Leg Hip
Flexion (Start)

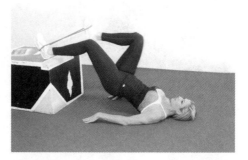

Static Elevated Bridge with Single Leg Hip
Flexion (End)

QUADRUPLED DONKEY KICKS

15 reps per side

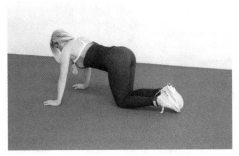

Quadrupled Donkey Kicks (Start)

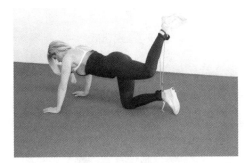

Quadrupled Donkey Kicks Basic (End)

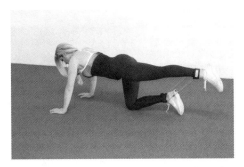

Quadrupled Donkey Kicks Advanced (End)

LIFT MORE THAN YOUR GROCERIES

"PIGEON" KICKBACKS

15 reps per side

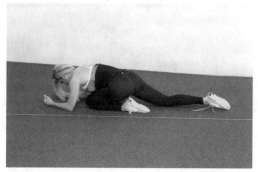

"Pigeon" Kickbacks Straight Leg (Start)

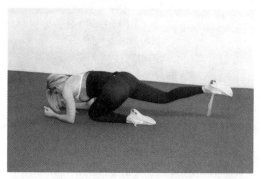

"Pigeon" Kickbacks Straight Leg (End)

LATERAL GLUTE STRENGTH – C1

90/90 hip abduction – 30 reps

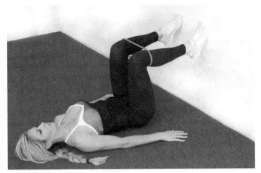

90/90 Hip Abduction (Start)

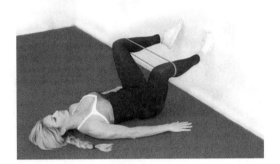

90-90 Hip Abduction (End)

LIFT MORE THAN YOUR GROCERIES

SIDE LYING "CLAMSHELL"
30 reps

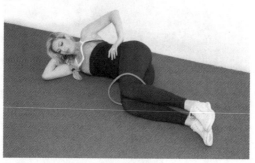

Side Lying "Clamshell" (Start)

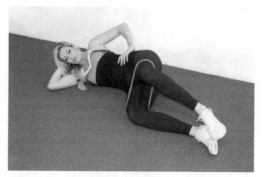

Side Lying "Clamshell" (End)

"BABY CRAWL"
15 reps per side

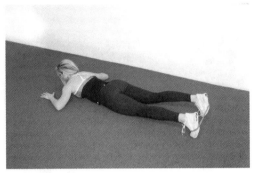

"Baby Crawl" (Start)

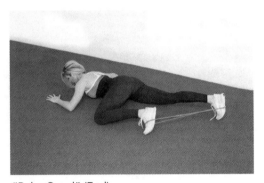

"Baby Crawl" (End)

CLAMSHELL TO SIDE PLANK

15 reps per side

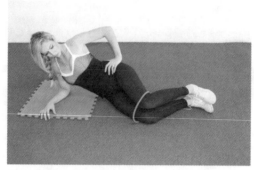

Clamshell to Side Plank (Start)

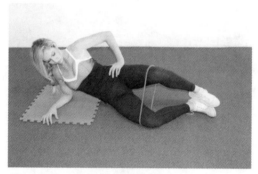

Clamshell to Side Plank (Middle)

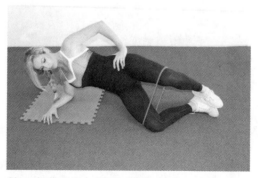

Clamshell to Side Plank (End)

◼ "FIRE HYDRANTS" ◼
15 reps per side

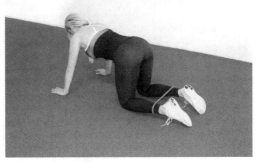

"Fire Hydrants" (Start)

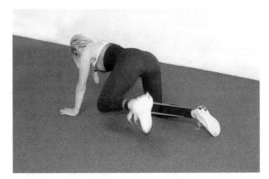

"Fire Hydrants" (End)

LIFT MORE THAN YOUR GROCERIES

CLAMSHELL TO SIDE PLANK HOLD

30 seconds per side

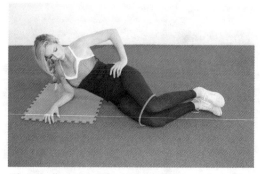

Clamshell to Side Plank Hold (End)

SIDE PLANK ABDUCTION (STRAIGHT LEG)

15 reps per side

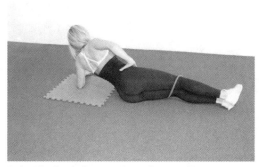

Side Plank Abduction Straight Leg (Start)

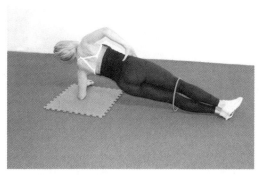

Side Plank Abduction Straight Leg (Middle)

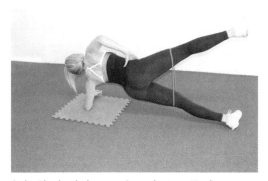

Side Plank Abduction Straight Leg (End)

LIFT MORE THAN YOUR GROCERIES

SIDE PLANK ABDUCTION HOLD (STRAIGHT LEG)

30 seconds per side

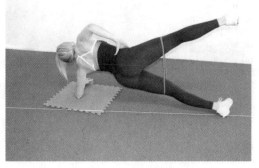

Side Plank Abduction Hold Straight Leg

PRONE ROTATIONAL DONKEY KICKS

30 reps

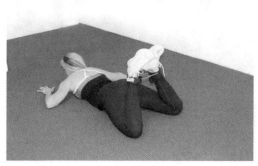

Prone Rotational Donkey Kicks (Start)

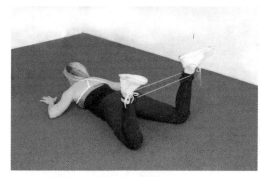

Prone Rotational Donkey Kicks (End)

LIFT MORE THAN YOUR GROCERIES

SUPINE PPT STRAIGHT LEG ABDUCTION

30 reps

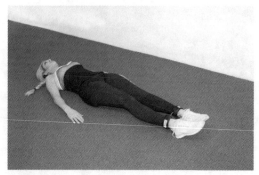

Supine PPT Straight Leg Abduction (Start)

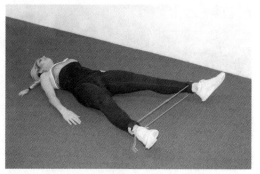

Supine PPT Straight Leg Abduction (End)

PRONE ROTATIONAL DONKEY KICK HOLD

30 seconds

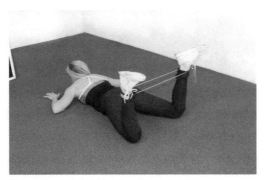

Prone Rotational Donkey Kick Hold

LIFT MORE THAN YOUR GROCERIES

▪ SUPINE PPT STRAIGHT LEG ABDUCTION HOLD ▪

30 seconds

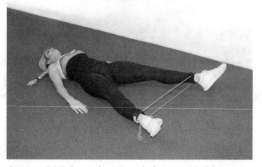

Supine PPT Straight Leg Abduction Hold

CHAPTER 10

Food Rules – Read and Digest

YOU'RE GON' LEARN TODAY

ONE OF THE reasons diet plans and programs fail so often is because they are just that: fixed and rigid. Giving people totally structured programs is disempowering much like giving a man a fish, instead of teaching him HOW to fish. It is disempowering. It is a temporary crutch that does little to address the underlying cause of the problem (case in point A: not knowing how to fish; case in point B: being stuck in the "old" diet paradigm). Some of the most popular programs will literally deliver EVERY meal and every calorie you're expected to consume on a given day. Not only is this a terrible idea, since eating a diet composed of 100% processed food is likely to lead to chronic problems; but more importantly, you'll never learn how to make your own healthy choices. Once you run out or can't afford the prepared meals anymore you're screwed.

Recipe books and conventional meal plans are equally disempowering. It's like being given all the right answers on a test: you may get a high score, but you never really learn anything. Just as the student will fail when the answers aren't whispered into her ear, the dieter will fail as soon as someone stops telling her exactly what to put in her mouth. Take my word on this; I have seen it happen again and again. Coddling and handholding DO NOT WORK. Unless you put your #biggirlpantson and make some serious changes, you will always end up back where you started.

The solution? It's definitely not having your food delivered or someone telling you exactly what to eat and/or cook at all times of the day. The solution is to learn how to do it for yourself, and more importantly understand WHY you should want to. Understanding the why is the sole obstacle between you and your goal of getting out of the vicious yo-yo cycle. I am not going to sugarcoat reality and feed you fluff like all the other diet books. And I am absolutely not going to dumb down my message or the science behind what we do. After all, where has that gotten you? I am going to teach you what you need to learn to effectively reach and maintain your goals for the rest of your life – without feeling deprived or stressed. It's a lot easier and much more fun than you think!

THE MEAT AND POTATOES

I will provide you with nutrition templates based on your body frame and phases of training, but by the end of the following chapters, you should fully understand WHY you are eating what you are eating and when.

It's time for a re-education about everything you thought you knew about food, nutrition, and dieting. It's time to learn how to fish.

WHY YOU WILL NEVER OUT-EXERCISE A ROTTEN DIET

We will start here because research study after research study show that *what you do nutritionally is the most important factor affecting body composition, fat loss, or muscle gain.* When most people make New Year's resolutions to lose a few pounds, the first thing they look at is their exercise habits. This is one of the biggest mistakes of our time.

A 1999 study on the effects of diet and different types of exercise on fat loss found:

"Overweight subjects were assigned to three groups: diet-only, diet plus aerobics, diet plus aerobics plus weights. The diet group lost 14.6 pounds of fat in 12 weeks. The diet plus aerobic group lost only one more pound (15.6 pounds) than the diet group (training was three times a week starting at 30 minutes and progressing to 50 minutes over the 12 weeks). The weight training group lost 21.1 pounds of fat (44% and 35% more than the diet and diet plus aerobic only groups respectively.

This study clearly shows that solid nutrition is the major factor in fat loss. Exercise (especially resistance training, as we've discussed) plays a role, but if you're not addressing what you put into your mouth, you're going to be spinning your gears. Another twelve-week study from 1986 also seems to agree:

"The obese women and men in the diet-only group (n=24) that reduced their caloric intake lost 5.5 kg and 8.4 kg, respectively. To achieve this degree of weight loss, women decreased their average caloric intake by 945 kilocalories a day while the men decreased their average intake by 1705 kilocalories a day. The exercise-only group (n = 24 obese men and women), performed a 30-minute walk/jog program 5 days/week. On average, the women expended 190 kilocalories per session while the men expended an average of 255 kilocalories per session, which resulted in a total weight loss of .6 kg and .3 kg for women and men, respectively. The women in the diet-only program decreased their body fat from 35% to 29%, whereas the women doing exercise only went from 35% to 33% body fat. Additionally, the men in the diet-only group decreased body fat from 26% to 21% whereas the exercise-only group experienced no change in their body fat)."

If you were reading the last study closely, you might have thought that it is not fair to compare dropping 945 calories a day through diet compared to burning 190 calories a day exercising. And you'd be right. It's not a fair comparison at all—and that's the point. The point is that there is *much* more you can do to impact how your nutrition affects your goals than simply exercise.

One of my favorite examples is the person who rewards himself after a workout in which he may have burned upwards of 600 calories (if he really crushed himself) by indulging in a "healthy" 1500 calorie milkshake aka smoothie. Don't laugh; post-workout sabotages are surprisingly pervasive. I used to run a fitness studio located right next to a smoothie shop, and I would see it all the time. To say it's frustrating watching your clients sabotage themselves is an understatement.

Now, none of this is to say that exercise doesn't matter. If you didn't sleepwalk through the last chapter, you should know by now that exercise is not optional. There is no one who has optimal levels of health AND looks great naked who doesn't exercise. But, you absolutely need to have the nutrition piece in place as well. The right type of exercise accelerates the fat loss of a sound nutrition plan. Not only that, when we're losing weight, exercise enables us to lose almost exclusively fat and keep our hard earned muscle—which is your goal if you want a Bikini Boss body. A good rule of thumb is that nutrition alone controls weight loss or weight gain which, remember, we don't really care about since we don't really care about the scale. (If you're suffering from scale amnesia, re-read the "Myths" section in chapter 6). The presence or absence of exercise, on the other hand, determines whether we gain or lose fat or muscle. It is important to not confuse the two. Our goal is to lose fat and build muscle, regardless of some arbitrary societal guidelines about what the numbers on a scale are supposed to say. If you want a lean, toned, and sculpted body, this is the way to do it!

FOOD QUANTITY – TOO MUCH VS. NOT ENOUGH

So far, we have determined that our nutrition matters A LOT. Let's talk about how to make it work in our favor. One of the biggest misconceptions in the nutritional world is the concept of calories in vs. calories out or, as I like to call it, the old paradigm. Many well-intentioned health professionals (including many medical doctors and nutritionists) still adhere to this dogma. We have been told for years if we eat 500 less calories a day for a week we will lose exactly one pound because one pound = 3500 calories. The biggest problem with this concept is it assumes our energy expenditure will remain constant. Unfortunately for this theory, human beings are not a closed system, nor does our metabolism take place in a research lab.

A recurring concept in the *Boss to Bikini* program is that fat loss and revving up the metabolism is not simply an issue of calories in vs. calories out. Fat loss IS, however, an issue of energy intake vs. energy expenditure. The key difference is "energy intake and expenditure" is dynamic while "calories in vs. calories out" is static. Our daily metabolism (energy expenditure) can fluctuate based on a variety of things, including our body weight, how long we exercise, what kind of exercise we do, our stress levels, which hormones are circulating, our sleep habits, and yes, even from our nutritional choices. What we eat, when we eat it, and how we combine different foods all have a different effect on how our bodies respond and how our body burns energy.

On the flip side of the coin, these same variables also impact our energy intake. The physiological state that we are in will change how we digest and absorb food and how we use different nutrients, vitamins, and minerals. For example, depending on when you eat carbohydrates they can either go directly to fueling your muscles or directly to the fat on the thighs. Something as simple as our breathing can impact the electrolyte balance within our body. Our hormonal fluctuations on a daily (and monthly) basis change what gets absorbed and what doesn't. The human body is incredibly complex with billions of complicated interactions occurring simultaneously. To expect it to behave like a machine just doesn't make sense.

We have already discussed the importance of nutrition on our body composition and health goals so let's talk about how much and what type of food we should be eating. Keep in mind, we will not be asking you to "count calories." It is neither productive, nor necessary. However, we do have to stick to a macronutrient range because if we are taking in too much food, it will surpass our energy expenditure no matter how hard we are training. The result would then be weight gain AND fat gain. On the other hand, not eating enough calories will be unproductive as well. Often, when women come to me frustrated with their lack of results, they're actually vastly undereating for their goals. We are going to make sure neither of the above happen. First things first.

LOSE FAT AND BUILD MUSCLE. CHOOSE ONE.

Building the body of your dreams comes down to two things: having more lean muscle and less excess body fat. Unfortunately, it's hard for most people to do both at the same time. There are three main scenarios when it's possible to achieve both simultaneously:

1. YOU HAVE A LOT OF FAT TO LOSE. When your body fat percentage is 40 percent or higher, it's possible to lose a LOT of fat and build muscle at the same time. When there is a lot of extra energy from excess fat, the body is much less likely to dip into your muscle for energy. This creates an environment where, despite massive fat loss, muscle can be built as well.

2. YOU'RE A TRUE BEGINNER. If you've never really lifted heavy weights (say a weight you couldn't lift more than ten times), or you've been weight lifting for less than six months, your muscles respond so favorably that even if you're in a deficit, your muscles will still grow. This is an extremely rare window where true body decomposition (turning "fat into muscle") can actually occur even in a caloric deficit.

3. YOU'RE ON STEROIDS. A dirty little secret in the fitness industry is that the use of steroids or other illegal performance enhancing drugs is surprisingly common. Many of the fitness models you see online or on TV only make money if their body looks a certain way. And because they're human, sometimes they'll fall off the wagon. To make sure such behavior doesn't cost them their livelihood, they'll often use any combination of drugs to help look a certain way, all year round. The rules of physiology change when you start putting artificial hormones into your system. These people can build muscle and lose fat at the same time, but given how harmful the steroids are to the body, it's just not worth it.

So, if you've been working out for a few years, aren't extremely overweight, aren't taking steroids but also don't have the body you're looking for, unfortunately, you're going to have to choose to work on one thing at a time—EITHER fat loss OR muscle gain. Our phase training workout programs are designed with this reality in mind. Aside from the situations listed above, the body is either in an anabolic mode (adding more stuff) or a catabolic mode (breaking stuff down). It's very rarely in both at the same time. You're EITHER building or breaking down so you need to figure out how to eat for both.

FOOD RULES – READ AND DIGEST

ON BUILDING MUSCLE

Muscle is metabolically expensive, so the body will only build it if there is good reason for doing so. This is why I often laugh when women think they will get huge lifting weights; it's just not that easy! You need the perfect storm for this to happen, which includes the right training frequency and intensity, and getting enough nutrients to support GROWTH. If you train hard without the nutrition to support it, nothing changes. If you take in enough calories to build muscle but don't train, you'll build… fat. Obviously, that's not our goal. Keep in mind, it's almost impossible (outside of the three scenarios above) to build muscle without building a little bit of fat. And that's okay. If you add five pounds of muscle to your frame and gain and incidental pound of fat, I PROMISE you, you'll be looking a lot better than before you started. Once again, I repeat, I am currently **FIFTEEN POUNDS** heavier than I was when I started working out the right way, and I look a million times better now. I love my body; I am no longer embarrassed to be in a bikini in front of people. I could have never gotten here had I been fixated on the scale. Muscle has mass, so if you're gaining it, the scale WILL go up. What you need to accept is that this isn't anything to fear; on the contrary, it's telling you everything is working as it should. THE ONLY REASON YOU ARE AFRAID TO GAIN WEIGHT IS BECAUSE YOU ARE CONDITIONED TO BE. But not anymore!

PATIENCE IS A VIRTUE

So, how much muscle can I build? This goes back to "Myth #4": Building muscle takes time. If you're looking for a quick fix you've failed already. Anyone you see with an amazing bikini body has been working hard and consistently for months, if not years. Studies on men show that in a drug-free environment, if they do everything perfectly, they can gain about one pound of muscle a month for about a year. Next training year would be half that. Next training year would be half that. After that, muscle gains are going to be pretty negligible. With hard training and a great nutrition plan, a guy might gain twenty to twenty-five pounds of muscle over three to four years!

Here comes the reality bitch slap. You're not a guy. Women can have up to FIFTEEN TIMES less testosterone then men. This hormonal difference means you can't gain muscles like the guys. Your body will only support about HALF of the gains that men can achieve. If you're a beginner, you might gain six pounds of muscle A YEAR. That's half a pound a month. That won't seem like a lot of changes on a day-to-day basis, but when you look at the big picture, six pounds of muscle is really a lot! Be patient, and those muscles will grow if you let them. You'll be shocked at how even the slightest growth can positively impact and help shape up your physique.

How much fat can I lose? Again, I'm going to consult "Myth 4." Noticing the trend? The good news is that fat loss rates are a lot faster than muscle building rates. Based on your body fat percentage, you can lose around one to three pounds of fat a WEEK. As a general rule, the more fat you have to lose, the faster you can lose it. If you're in that 40 percent or higher body fat bracket, two to three pounds a week is possible. On average, however, you can lose about one pound a week if you're doing most things right. A few too many cheat meals and a few too many missed workouts, of course, will slow things down. And, of course, the leaner you are, the harder it is (both nutritionally and exercise-wise) to lose fat. At a certain level of leanness (six pack abs, with visible ab veins), you may only be able to lose 0.25-0.5 pounds of fat per week This shouldn't apply to you unless you plan to do a fitness competition since you won't need to be that lean. For most lifestyle clients who adhere to the program you'll know you're on track if you're losing an average of one pound of fat per week.

DO NOT FALL INTO THIS QUICKSAND

Many women unfortunately get frustrated when they don't see fat loss rates occur faster. It's not surprising that these women are typically the same people obsessed with the numbers on the scale. "I only lost two pounds this week" is parroted far too often early on by women in our programs. It's a sad fact but some of them do not have the patience or foresight to see the program to the end. For some, it is just too difficult to get out of the weight loss mentality. We often laugh because 99 percent of the time, we see these same girls jumping from program to program with no results to show. There is no such thing as a quick fix, ladies! Not trusting the process and expecting immediate results is the biggest trap women fall into. Do yourself a favor and don't let this be you.

IT'S NOT ALL ABOUT THE SCALE

Two pounds a week would still be 104 pounds lost in a year! If you are morbidly obese, you would still be happy if you're losing more than 100 pounds in a year. Even half a pound a week is a 26-pound annual fat loss; that's something to be proud of. Let's get real.

Another thing to keep in mind is water fluctuations. Based on how many carbs you eat on a given day (carbs are stored in the muscle with water), your hydration levels, and where you are in your menstrual cycle (let's face it, how many of us know we're on our cycle when we start feeling bloated), your scale weight can fluctuate as much as ten pounds! It's impossible to gain or lose five pounds in a day from muscle or fat, but it's actually pretty easy to have that big of a change from water weight. That's another reason to NOT base results on what the scale is doing.

Still want a quick fix?

Let's take a look at what actually happens when you crash diet.

The landmark study on prolonged starvation diets was conducted by the University of Minnesota in the 1950s. People were put on a diet of about half of their daily maintenance nutrition for a period of six months. Sure, people lost weight but keeping people on a low calorie plan for that long a period of time created a nasty list of side effects including:

- An insatiable appetite for months after being reintroduced to normal food
- A significant drop in physical endurance
- Decreases in strength
- Diminished reflexes
- Lowered heart volume
- Impaired concentration
- Poor judgment in aptitude tests
- Reduced sexual performance AND interest
- Excess nervousness and anxiety
- General apathy towards life
- Depression
- An obsession with food
- Accelerated aging

These are obviously terrible side effects, and nothing justifies putting yourself through this on purpose, especially when there are more effective and easier ways to accomplish your goals. You think waiting a few months for results is hard? Try living for months, if not years with the aforementioned symptoms and unable to burn fat no matter what you do. If you think it can't happen to you, think again! Every day, we see women in our programs who have had their metabolisms DESTROYED by trainers and/or coaches who put them on extremely low calorie diets for months. I've seen it take more than a year of proper eating to get their hormones back in balance. Going through this is not only unnecessary for fat loss, but is extremely dangerous and absolutely not worth it.

SO AM I BUILDING? OR LEANING?

We've just discussed that the majority of people must choose one option. That's why we have set up our plans and phases as EITHER leaning OR building/maintenance. The reason we put building and maintenance in the same category is that the nutritional surplus that you need to build muscle (at the high end, half a pound a month) is pretty negligible over maintenance if you're training properly.

Fully hydrated human skeletal muscle is no more than 15 to 20 percent protein, 4 to 8 percent fat and minimal glycogen. The rest is water (about 80 percent) and minerals. Despite what many people believe, it just doesn't take that much extra per day to build muscle, 800-1000 calories per pound MAX. If we look at half a pound of muscle gain a month, that's 400 to 500 extra calories a MONTH, or an extra thirteen to sixteen calories A DAY. That is nearly impossible to measure. As such, maintenance and building is pretty much the same thing nutritionally as long as you're in a consistent training program at a relatively difficult intensity.

BEHIND THE SCENES—HOW THE PROGRAM IS DESIGNED

The nutrition plans we've devised are based on metabolic formulas to help facilitate your fat loss, muscle building, and metabolism-revving goals. The following sections show how we designed your programs. Some of you may not be interested in this behind-the-scenes information but I know that some of you Type-As want to understand the "why" behind our recommendations.

The numbers for both fat loss and muscle building are based off a variety of metabolic calculators including the Harris-Benedict, the Katch-McArdle, and the Cunningham equations. The numbers are also based on recommendations from dozens of the world's top health and fitness professionals. There are several formulas for daily caloric intake, and many factor in weight, height, activity level, etc. Most are extremely complicated. But at the end of the day, they all usually end up right around the same place.

For fat loss—Our goal is to find the nutritional "sweet spot" where you lose fat, but don't lose muscle. Too big of a deficit will decrease your metabolism, thus decreasing your energy expenditure, which is not going to help you hit your fat-loss goals.

For muscle building—At the high end, our goal is to find the "sweet spot" where you gain muscle, but not fat. Too much of a surplus and you'll still build muscle, but you'll build excess fat too. If I had to choose, I'd pick building muscle WITHOUT fat.

FOOD QUALITY, AND TRAFFIC LIGHTS

Health always comes first

Any nutritional plan should promote health. When we say health, we will use the World Health Organization definition: "Health is a state of complete physical, mental and social well-being and not merely the absence of disease or infirmity." Health is everything working right, which is not the same as not feeling like something is wrong. Until blood pressure screenings became commonplace, the first symptom of heart disease used to be a heart attack. Hypertension, diabetes, and various types of cancer are a few examples of diseases that often advance far before we have any symptoms. How we feel is quite honestly a terrible measure of how healthy we are.

Consequently, you can understand why health should be a primary concern in every nutrition plan. This seems obvious, but given the rise of "smoothie-diets," "cookie-diets," "juice-diets," etc., it clearly needs to be discussed. **Any diet that excludes foods that have nutrients that are essential for human survival should be avoided.** The *Boss to Bikini* nutritional philosophy is designed to give you a full array of carbohydrates, proteins, fats, vitamins, minerals, fiber, and all of the things your body needs to run properly. We will NEVER expect you to pursue fat loss in exchange for your health. You can have both—and you will have both! In fact, one of the most common and fulfilling things I hear when women start our program is how great they FEEL. That they look better is a given but they are always pleasantly surprised at how amazing they feel. Mark my words—you will become addicted to THAT feeling.

The "bread and butter" (pun intended since we don't eat bread)) of this program is based in anthropology and evolutionary biology. It is based on the foods that our species has been eating for long periods of time, making them the foods our body metabolizes most efficiently. It is a very 'nutritionally dense' program, and you will learn how to get many more vitamins, nutrients, and fiber than most other programs.

Because of its balanced nature, this program is sustainable for the REST OF YOUR LIFE. The previous statement warrants re-stating: **this program is sustainable for the rest of your life.** Its principles have been used everywhere, from helping people lose a few extra pounds of body weight, getting people a Bikini Fitness stage-ready body, and helping world-class athletes win

gold medals. It is the most innate type of diet and nutrition and when we start eating the way our bodies are designed, the results are nothing short of amazing.

THE GOOD, THE BAD AND THE UGLY

The *Boss to Bikini* nutritional program is a natural food-based program designed to optimize health and body composition. We will provide you with the actual macronutrient portions or "how much to eat" on our meal plans later in the chapter but the fundamentals of the *"what to eat"* part are summarized below:

GREEN LIGHT
- Vegetables
- Natural, Unprocessed Meats (animal protein, fish, eggs)
- Fruits
- Proceed freely

These are the foods that should make up the majority of your daily content, ideally 100 percent.

> I am not encouraging you to eat only fruit all day every day. I am saying these foods are the most ideal choices to use to fill your macronutrient amounts on your meal plan.

Our genes are optimized for this kind of eating, and if these foods make up the

116

majority of your diet, you will never need to worry about getting enough protein, healthy fats, vitamins, minerals, or fiber. A good rule of thumb is whether you could eat the food raw, as it exists in nature, without any processing. If it can be bought on the perimeter of grocery stores it's typically ideal. This type of eating will also help make you "chronic disease proof," as the majority of chronic diseases are directly caused or exacerbated by poor nutritional choices. While eating these foods 100 percent of the time is ideal, we understand that some people will want to transition more gradually into their new lifestyle, and that we also need to allow some flexibility for life as well. As such, we will give you a range and say that 80 to 100 percent of your daily calories should come from these choices. Just remember, the more you choose poorly processed, nutrient deficient foods, the more challenging it will be to simultaneously reach your body composition and health goals.

YELLOW LIGHT

- Rice (white and brown)
- Potatoes (white, red and sweet)
- Quinoa
- Nuts and seeds
- Protein powders
  Proceed—with some caution

These foods can make up a significant part of your nutrition program, depending on your goals and your lifestyle. However, none of these things are actually **necessary** for optimal health or a perfect looking body. Depending on your fitness goals, it may be beneficial to incorporate these in addition to fruits and vegetables. For example: a yoga instructor who has never lifted a weight in her life and eats a vegetarian diet does not need to increase her calorie and carbohydrate numbers any higher because she's most likely getting enough carbohydrates from the fruits, veggies, nuts, and seeds she's eating. In addition, most likely she isn't participating in any high intensity, glycogen depleting activities and her energy expenditure is not high enough to warrant these foods. Conversely, a Bikini Fitness athlete or endurance runner may absolutely need to add in some additional carbohydrates from these sources as part of her daily carbohydrate intake to help replace glycogen stores and avoid muscle loss.

Nuts and Seeds

Nuts and seeds fit in this category because while they are healthy and fully natural, they should not be used too frequently. They are extremely calorically dense (which can easily put you over your daily macronutrient numbers). They are a much better snack than a bag of cookies, but too much of a good thing can always become a problem. Vegetarians, however, are an exception to this rule. While the body is optimized to utilize the amino acids in animal proteins (animal proteins have a more complete complement of essential amino acids), nuts and seeds can be used as a primary protein source in the rotation for people who don't eat animal products. If you use nuts as a protein source you must also count the fat and carbohydrates involved as well.

The security blanket of "Clean Eating"

Many nutritional gurus who take the "eat as much as you want as long as it's clean" approach grossly underestimate how much some people will actually eat. They say "as long as you're eating clean, your body will respond." I hate to break it to you, but this isn't always true. It's especially not true for calorically dense foods like nuts, oils, and dried fruits. Even though these foods are totally healthy, it is easy to overeat them, so be cautious when you're eating these foods.

Rice and Potatoes

Higher density carbohydrate sources like potatoes and rice can be used by certain athletes or clients who have higher training loads to increase performance and/or aesthetic results. They are not necessary for survival or to get body composition results for most people; however, depending on your goals, they can constitute a good portion of your diet.

Meal Replacements & Protein Powders

Liquid calories (meal replacements and protein powders) can be used in three situations:

1. When women have a difficult time going from the old paradigm way of eating, i.e., barely anything all day to the new paradigm way of eating, i.e., frequently and a lot. It is sometimes a hard transition for women and they have a difficult time adjusting to eating this volume of food. Incorporating a shake or two a day helps tremendously and allows them to get used to this type of eating schedule.

2. During times of laziness. I don't mean to insult you but we're all so busy that occasionally, we get lazy. But the reality is that few people have a lifestyle SO demanding that they cannot make the time to prepare their own healthy meals. Case in point: It only takes two or three minutes to scramble up some eggs. Most nutritionally successful people prepare the majority of their meals in advance on a day or two of the week when they have some free time. In fitness, we call this "meal prep" days. This makes it much easier to stay healthy and on track on days where there is less disposable time. However, we get it. We understand sometimes you are pressed for time and don't have optimal health choices at your disposal. In these circumstances, having a default healthy

118

product like a quality protein shake is a lot better than a breakfast at Starbucks or a lunch at McDonalds.

3. As a supplement for people having a difficult time hitting the protein goals because the volume of food isn't enough. Considering none of us are male body builders, I don't see this being an issue.

RED LIGHT
(Danger approaching)
- Refined sugar
- Trans fats
- Dairy
- Most grains
- Caffeine
- Alcohol

These are the foods and products that that have no nutritional value at all, or the pros are heavily outweighed by the cons. **With any red light food product, moderation is encouraged.**

Refined Sugar
Despite Americans steadily decreasing their animal fat (saturated fat) intake over the last thirty years, obesity rates have continued to increase. One thing that has increased almost in line with obesity rates is sugar consumption. Very simply: added sugar makes you fat. Even fruit juice consumption promotes obesity, as the lack of fiber makes it much easier to take in very high sugar intake. To put it in the simplest

terms, sugar blocks fat loss. It tells the body you have fuel coming to use as energy so there is no need to tap into our energy stores (fat).

Added sugars also promote inflammation, which is linked to the development of every chronic disease there is. Dr. Robert Lustig, a pediatric endocrinologist from UCSF, goes so far to say that added sugars are poisons, and should be regulated as strictly as alcohol. Discussing the diversity of negative metabolic effects of high refined sugar intakes is beyond the scope of this book, but Dr. Lustig gives a brilliant lecture on the dangers of sugar consumption (easily searchable on YouTube) called "Sugar: The Bitter Truth." It is worth ninety minutes of your time to learn why sugar should be used as little as possible.

Trans Fats & Pro-inflammatory Fats
Artificially made trans fats cannot be recognized by the body as food and as such, are a toxin. Many U.S. restaurants and even some countries, including Switzerland and Denmark, have banned trans fats. Trans fats have been linked to Alzheimer's disease, cancer, diabetes, liver dysfunction, depression, infertility, and of course, obesity. Trans fats are created by chemically adding hydrogen groups to vegetable oils, which makes them less likely to spoil. Anytime you read "partially hydrogenated" on an ingredient label trans fats are present. The most common foods with trans fats include

119

margarine, shortening, most processed and frozen foods (this includes numerous kids' snacks!), and almost everything commercially deep fried. And forget about the overly processed protein bars you see in convenience and grocery stores; they are full of trans fats too.

Trans fat = shit storm

Furthermore, trans fats are extremely inflammatory—notice the trend here? When choosing fats and oils, we should only use oils that are closest to their natural state. Just imagine what types of twisted processes must occur to extract large volumes of oil from a grain.

Oils to avoid:
- Canola
- Soybean
- Corn
- Flaxseed
- Peanut
- Sunflower seed
- Safflower, cottonseed
- Grapeseed oils

Oils that get the green light include
- Coconut oil
- MCT (Medium-Chain Triglycerides) oil
- Olive oil
- Avocado oil
- Fish oil (omega-3)

Dairy Products

Are you ready to be grossed out? WE ARE THE ONLY SPECIES THAT DRINKS ANOTHER SPECIES' MILK. Think about this for second. Do you see monkeys drinking lion's milk or horses drinking milk from a sheep? It's not natural! Species produce milk to feed their young until they are independent or advanced enough to eat on their own. Mother's milk provides nutrients and immunoglobulins to offspring to ensure survival of their species. Milk, of any kind, is not necessary for humans after weaning. The fallacy that we need to drink milk for calcium is perpetuated by the dairy industry. It's just not the truth! All the nutrients we need from dairy can be easily acquired through plant sources. These alternative sources are even more effective because drinking milk actually causes the body to leach calcium from our bones.

From an evolutionary standpoint, it would have been impossible to drink large amounts of milk before the domestication of livestock. Our genes evolved more than 50,000 years ago; agriculture and livestock have been around a lot less, meaning dairy could never have been a staple of our diet. To quote an article from the *American Journal of Clinical Nutrition* on the myths of the health importance of dairy:

> *Although cow milk has been widely recommended in Western countries as necessary for growth and bone health, evidence collected during the past 20*

years shows the need to rethink strategies for building and maintaining strong bones. Osteoporotic bone fracture rates are highest in countries that consume the most dairy, calcium, and animal protein. Most studies of fracture risk provide little or no evidence that milk or other dairy products benefit bone. Accumulating evidence shows that consuming milk or dairy products may contribute to the risk of prostate and ovarian cancers, autoimmune diseases, and some childhood ailments.

Depending on your ethnic background, you may be even more likely to not tolerate dairy products. Some 95 percent of Asian Americans, 74 percent of Native Americans, 70 percent of African Americans, 53 percent of Mexican-Americans, and 15 percent of Caucasians have been shown to have lactose intolerance. If we examine some of the other allergenic proteins in milk, up to 60 percent of all individuals may have an inability to process dairy to some degree. Whether because of a true allergy, lactose intolerance, or other physiologic process, dairy is not an optimal nutrition choice for the majority of people.

Most people simply feel better when they remove dairy from their diets, and we recommend using dairy sparingly, if at all. There are plenty of alternatives such as almond and coconut milk which taste great and don't have the negative and inflammatory effects of cow's milk.

Caffeine

Caffeine has gotten mixed reviews in the literature regarding its potential health effects. On the positive side, it has been found to improve performance in both sprint and endurance sports, can be a potent antioxidant, and as we all know, increases mental alertness. On the negative side, let's state the obvious: It is an addictive drug. A large majority of people around the world suffer from some sort of caffeine dependency. I mean, the advent of Starbucks has made super strong coffee easily accessible and created more crazed coffee fanatics than ever before. And while I, too, am guilty of this addiction, here's where I really get concerned. Caffeine is a central nervous system stimulant which over stimulates the adrenal glands to produce epinephrine (adrenaline) and cortisol. Normally, the body is only designed to stay in a state of stress physiology for a few minutes (refer back to "fight or flight"), but caffeine has a half-life of ninety minutes to nine and one-half hours, which keeps those hormones elevated for extended periods of time.

While our body is in a stress physiology (elevated epinephrine and cortisol levels), many bad things happen that slow down our quest to lose body fat. Though I've dedicated an entire chapter to stress physiology previously, it's important enough to bring up again.

The Stress Factor

The impact of stress on body physiology is well documented. Despite this fact, far too few people acknowledge that getting their stress levels under control can be the missing link to hitting their health and body composition goals. In addition to caffeine, many other factors keep the stress hormones elevated, including systemic inflammation, environmental toxins, very low calorie diets, excessive exercise, and sleep deprivation. One of my favorite quotes on sleep deprivation and its impact on body composition comes from Robb Wolf, author of The Paleo Solution.

> *"Inadequate sleep cock-blocks fat loss."*

In addition, chronically elevated stress hormones cause us to crave food sources that rapidly convert into energy (think sugary snacks), elevate blood sugar, give our bodies signals to deposit abdominal fat, increase free radicals in the body, raise blood pressure, decrease immune function and tissue repair, and elevate blood cholesterol levels.

While you're working on kicking your caffeine habit, work on eliminating the other stressors from your life, too. Your body will thank you.

Alcohol

We're not going to dive too deeply into why to stay away from alcohol, because you already know why it is not going to help you reach your goals. It is a central nervous system depressant, provides calories without any nutritional value, is catabolic to muscle (breaks it down) and the list of all the other negative physiological side effects is almost endless. A glass or two of wine per week won't kill you but remember you can crawl or sprint to your goals. Zero is optimal.

Disclaimer: Everything in moderation.

Back to Myth #2 (you have to be perfect all of the time), you don't have to give up alcohol to get a rockin' body. A crazy night of partying every few weeks isn't going to totally derail your goals. It just isn't going to help. So enjoy your birthdays, weddings, graduations, holiday parties, etc., but get back on the wagon once the celebration is over.

Grains and Legumes

I saved this for the end of the "red light" section because most people have an unnatural love affair with grain products. Many people can easily give up coffee, alcohol, candy—hell, even sex—for a few days, but ask these same people to go a day or two without bread or pasta, and you might think they were asked to murder their first born. Whether we're talking about bread, pasta, cookies, cakes, pizza or beer, grain products are a staple for most people. They are also keeping most people from reaching their health and body composition goals. For some, grains may even unknowingly kill them.

Some of the more progressive researchers and doctors who care about nutrition have supported the idea that gluten (a highly inflammatory protein found most notably in wheat, rye, and barley) is not the best choice for most people. There are many drawbacks from gut irritation, increased insulin resistance, bloating, decreased intestinal absorption, and a laundry list of others. The biggest problem with grains though, is that gluten is not the only culprit.

There are proteins in every grain and legume that affect the physiology in a similar manner to gluten. Almost everyone (yes, even those without true Celiac disease) will have improved blood chemistry, feel better, and look better upon removing grains from the diet.

Note: Rice was introduced earlier as an acceptable choice for some people (especially endurance athletes), depending on their performance goals. Yes, we know that rice is a grain. Of all the grain products, however, white rice seems to cause the fewest problems. We promote white rice over brown rice, because the bran (the outer covering of the grain that makes it brown) contains

a variety of anti-nutrients that negate the benefits of the extra vitamins and minerals. Adding vitamins and minerals is useless if you create a terrible physiological state in the body by doing so.

GRAINS AND LEGUMES TO AVOID:
- Wheat (white, whole or sprouted)
- Peas
- Beans (any and all)
- Peanuts
- Soy Beans

One of the biggest adjustments you'll make with the *Boss to Bikini* program is learning that grains don't have to be a staple of your diet. We have had numerous clients over the years show radical changes in their health by removing grains, even among those who didn't have a true Celiac disease. Getting rid of highly inflammatory products can help by decreasing bloating, reducing headaches and menstrual cramps, and improving mental clarity. To help you better understand the deleterious effects that grains have on the body, I suggest you read three books that focus in detail on the physiology behind why we should ideally give them up. You'll get a much better explanation from these books.

- **THE PALEO SOLUTION:** The Original Human Diet by Robb Wolf (Victory Belt Publishing)

- **THE PRIMAL BLUEPRINT:** Reprogram your genes for effortless weight loss, vibrant health, and boundless energy by Mark Sisson (Primal Nutrition, Inc.)
- **THE PALEO DIET:** Lose Weight and Get Healthy by Eating the Foods You Were Designed to Eat by Loren Cordain (Wiley)

Before you freak out—NO, we are not promoting a strict Paleo diet. Our philosophy on health and nutrition is, however, built on the ideal way to eat and move based on evolutionary biology and Paleo proponents have similar views to this approach. While I don't agree that eating an exclusively Paleo diet is ideal for everyone (remember, everyone's physiology is different and some are better adapted for fats and carbs) I do feel these experts' stance on eliminating grains is accurate and highly beneficial for most individuals.

There is nothing, nutritionally speaking, in grains that you can't get from fruits and vegetables. And fruits and veggies deliver the nutrients without any of those terrible side effects. Remove grains from your diet, and watch your health and body make a turn for the better.

If you've noticed, it was much easier to explain the "Green Light" section than the "Red Light" section. Most people intuitively know what the healthiest food choices are: vegetables, meats and fruits. It's when we make excuses for deviating

from these basics that we have a difficult time reaching our goals. When we stop blindly following programs and recommendations, and understand exactly WHY to make a specific nutritional choice, magic happens.

DIVIDE AND CONQUER: PROTEINS, CARBS, AND FATS (OH MY!)

Every process that the body uses to run itself is based on how it is fueled. Nutritionally, this generally comes down to water, vitamins, minerals, proteins, fats, and carbohydrates. The proper function of every cell and every reaction all comes back to proper nutrition. To better understand why we make certain recommendations, you first need to understand how the major macronutrients—protein, carbohydrates, and fat—work within the body.

WHAT ARE MACRONUTRIENTS?

Macronutrients are molecules that can be converted and used for energy by the body. They include carbohydrates, protein, and fats. Their primary role is to provide energy but their secondary role depends on the specific macronutrient. Carbohydrates are the main delivery system for vitamins and minerals (through fruits and vegetables). Fats play a critical role in cell structure and nerve function. In addition to the ability to be used for fuel, proteins are the main building blocks for almost ALL of the cellular components of our body.

Now that we have discussed what foods to choose and how much you'll be eating, let's move on to how to combine things. With regard to the macronutrients, we are going to start and pay the most attention to protein and here's why:

1. Carbohydrate tolerance varies widely. Our body can tolerate very high levels AND very low levels (a nutritional state called ketosis). Our body can functionally make carbohydrates from the building blocks of protein and fat. They are also the main delivery system for vitamins and minerals, and are the preferred energy source for the brain, but they are not essential for the body as an energy source. While most athletes (yourself included) need them to function properly, they still are not essential for survival. Keep in mind, though, surviving and thriving are two different things. While you don't NEED a lot of carbs, most of you will feel and look better by including them in your diet.

2. Fat intake can vary widely. At the low end, if fat intake is 15 percent or less of your diet, you start to have some nasty side effects (very similar to what was seen in the Minnesota starvation experiment). At the high end, there are some populations, such as the Intuit, who get between 80 and 90 percent of their daily calories from fat.

PROTEINS

Protein requirements are much more critical, and are the least variable of the macronutrients with respect to how much you need. The U.S. Department of Agriculture recommendations for daily protein intake to avoid deficiency are 46 grams for adult women and 56 grams for adult men.

If this amount of protein seems like a trivial amount, that's because it is. These numbers do not take into account body size or activity level and, in my opinion, even for sedentary people they are probably too low. Let's also remember that avoiding deficiency is NOT our goal. Optimizing health and body composition is our focus. Many experts agree with me, so let's figure out what OPTIMAL protein intakes should be if you want to hit your goals.

All numbers are in grams per pound of total body weight.

Dieticians of Canada: 0.5-0.8

American Dieticians Association: 0.5-0.8

American College of Sports Medicine: 0.5-0.8

National Sports and Conditioning Association: 0.7-0.9

Now let's look at what some of the world's leading sports nutrition gurus say.

Many nutrition leaders not mentioned below base protein recommendations on percentages of total calories. I'll discuss later why this thinking is flawed, and as such I only referenced those who used protein recommendations based on body weight.

All numbers are in grams per pound of total body weight.

Craig Ballantyne: 1.0 lb.

John Berardi: 0.6-0.9 lb. (1.0-1.5 lb. for bodybuilders)

Alwyn Cosgrove: 1lb. (1.0 lb. of lean body mass for cutting to lower overall calories)

Lyle McDonald: 0.7-0.9 lb. for endurance athletes, 1.0-1.5 lb. for power & strength athletes)

Charles Poliquin: "about" 1.0 lb., up to 2 lb. for bodybuilders

Mark Sisson: 0.7-1.0 lb.

Tom Venuto: 1.0 lb. (1.5 lb. for bodybuilders or figure athletes entering a contest)

Robb Wolf: 0.7-1.0 lb.

Alan Aragon: 0.6-0.7 lb.

Generally put the national associations recommend a little less, while the people who make their living off of client results recommend a little more. *I'd* prefer to err on the side of a little too much protein because too little protein can limit or sacrifice performance and/or results, but too much just becomes a more expensive source of calories. Trust me I know that organic meat is not cheap!

Based on what has been discussed, *the Boss to Bikini* programs include **0.5-1.0 of protein per pound of desired body weight.** Many research studies show that there is no measurable benefit in muscle gain by going over 1g per pound.

The best sources for dietary protein are natural meats (for the purposes of this discussion, eggs and fish are also meat). There have never been and there never will be healthy sedentary populations, and on this program, you will be exercising. Exercising bodies need protein to fuel their muscles. Once again, we recommend 0.5g-1.0g of protein per pound of IDEAL body weight. (Example: If you are 200 pounds but would like to be 150 pounds, our plans will recommend 75 to 150 grams/day). Animals providing unprocessed meats fed their most natural diet in their most natural habitat are the best options but slightly processed foods (canned tuna, protein powders, deli meats) get the yellow light.

I have not listed any protein recommendations based on percentages of total calories because protein requirements are based primarily on the amount of lean muscle mass you carry, not how much you're eating. Whether you're 5'2" and 115 pounds or 5'2" and 175 pounds, your protein requirements don't really change. However, your carbohydrate and fat numbers might.

CARBOHYDRATES AND FATS

Let's move on to the fun (and usually emotional) stuff—carbohydrates, or "carbs" and fat. If we go back to our first recommendation of eating real food, by simply eating the required amount of protein (read: meat) per day for your body type, and use the right essential fatty acid supplements, you'll automatically consume enough fat for optimal health. It becomes a little more difficult if you're a vegan, but I'll discuss how to properly add fat later, and it is quite easy to get a decent amount of healthy fats in your diet.

So far we have determined optimal protein amounts and these amounts will also give us an appropriate amount of fat (i.e., whole eggs and 90 percent lean ground beef both get 50 percent of their calories from fat). However, we are probably still way behind our daily caloric requirements. We also haven't touched vitamins and minerals. Here's where carbs and fats come in.

It is important to note that there are several very healthy societies that support both high carb and low carb options. There are Inuit and African societies that consistently get the majority of their calories from fat, and there are Asian societies that get 70 percent or more of their calories from carbohydrates. From a health standpoint, either could work fine. But if your goals are to be healthy AND have a sexy bikini body, moderate levels of proteins, carbohydrates, AND fats will be our optimal situation. The reasons come down to ***compliance***.

The explanations for whys diets fail are **ALWAYS** issues of compliance. Some nutritional protocols are simply more difficult to follow than others. Anything that does not leave you satisfied or is too difficult to fit into your lifestyle will ultimately fail you. There are hormones responsible for feeling full (satiety), and they are activated in much higher levels from diets high in fat or protein, than from diets high in carbohydrates. All other things being equal, **the nutrition plan that has best compliance will get the best results.**

The Boss to Bikini carb recommendations are based on not just fueling muscles, but promoting compliance. Most people do not function well on extremely low carb or ketogenic diets (<20g of carbohydrates per day), so we will not suggest ZERO carbs.

Depending on the phase you're in, you'll also be eating different carb amounts, too. Since the maintenance and building phases are higher in calories, they will obviously be higher in carbs as well.

We will recommend an amount of carbohydrate that promotes maximum volume, and maximum nutrient density while minimizing calories. This amount is 100-150 grams per day. How much is 100-150g of carbohydrate? In the grain world, not much. Two cups of cooked rice or oatmeal is about 100g. In the fruit and vegetable world, you get a whole lot more to eat.

One POUND of spinach is only fifteen

grams of carbohydrate and 100 calories. A pound of frozen vegetables is twenty grams and 150 calories. If you've ever tried to eat a pound of spinach in one day, you know it is a LOT of food. If you're eating a pound of vegetables a day, anyone who suggests your diet is unhealthy deserves a punch in the face. One pound of veggies contains ridiculous amounts of vitamins and minerals. Vegetables are your best friend in your quest towards sustainable health, and looking great. To maximize food volume (volume = more filling which helps with compliance), I suggest eating as many vegetables as you can.

Regarding fruit, after crunching some numbers, I have found that an average piece of "hand" fruit is about 25 grams of carbohydrate (a banana, apple, peach, etc.). Once again, since compliance is our golden rule, let's optimize our fruit intake to promote less hunger and maximum nutritional benefit. **We will do this by timing our fruit intake around workouts. I'll explain more later, but for now, if you're going to eat fruit, do it as part of your pre-workout or post-workout meals.**

For most of you, 100-150g of carbohydrates will support your health, help optimize your body composition, and even allow you to perform athletically at a fairly high level. Unless you're a professional endurance athlete, this level of carbohydrate should be fine.

The Meal Frequency Myth

One of the first things regarding weight loss you are likely to hear from doctors, nutritionists and trainers is that you have to eat four to six meals a day to help with your fat loss efforts. They say doing so helps keep hunger at bay, and helps rev your metabolism. BUT DOES IT?

To quote a 1997 study from the British Journal of Nutrition on the validity of these claims:

"There is no evidence that weight loss on hypo-energetic regimens is altered by meal frequency." Here is another quote on the topic from a research article:

"If eating more frequently makes it easier to control/reduce calories, it will help you to lose weight/fat. If eating more frequently makes it harder to control/reduce calories, or makes you eat more, you will gain weight. If eating less frequently makes it harder for you to control/reduce calories (because you get hungry and binge), it will hurt your efforts to lose weight/fat. If eating less frequently makes it easier to control/reduce calories (for any number of reasons), then that will help your efforts to lose weight/fat)."

It really comes down to personal preference. If you get better results from eating just two or three times a day, that's what you should do. If you get better results from eating 10 meals a day, that's what you should do (as well as investing in stock in Tupperware). At the end of the day, as long as your macronutrient goals are being hit, there is no difference how you hit them.

HOWEVER… We recommend higher meal frequencies for the reasons described in this excerpt from an Instagram post I made awhile back about this topic:

"Whether you're eating two or three times a day or five to seven times a day, in the end what matters most is your CALORIES and MACROS."

BENEFITS OF EATING MORE FREQUENTLY

Eating four to seven small meals is ideal for some people. In fact, I personally eat smaller meals more frequently and recommend my girls do and I feel it's advantageous for most people to do so as well. Here are the reasons:

- When you are in an intense training program designed to build your body and burn fat it requires a lot of food. Splitting the meals up throughout the day makes it easier to get all the food in without feeling stuffed and bloated.
- For some people (like me) going long periods without food tends to make them more ravenous and more likely to overeat.
- For some, intense training and physiological stress can impair digestion and cause lack of digestive enzymes to be released and subsequently lead to poor digestion and assimilation. Eating smaller meals allows the digestive system to work more efficiently. And yes intense training is a physiological stress to the body.

Research has shown a correlation between less frequent protein intake (leucine, specifically) and muscle wasting. Although there are nutritional supplements that help avoid this problem, it becomes a non-issue with increased meal frequency.

So when we look at what's best for overall aesthetic results, while it is the total calories and macros which matter most, you definitely need to take into account the benefits listed above. What works for one person may not for another.

It all comes down to what makes you, the client, most compliant.

129

BACK TO THE BASICS

So we have covered how we set up your protein intake **(0.5-1.0g/pound/day)** and carbohydrate intake **(100—150g/day)**. The problem here is that this is not a whole lot of calories. If we take a 125-pound female and put her at the mid-range of the protein requirements and give her 100 grams of carbs, we are left with about ninety-four grams of protein. That amount of protein combined with the carbs comes out to 775 calories (400 from carbs and 375 from protein). This would be near "starvation" numbers and we already know what happens with starvation. Let's talk about filling the void.

The numbers in my example are a little flawed, because there are no meat sources that are 100 percent protein. Even an extra lean chicken breast has a few grams of fat. A whole egg gets about half its calories from fat and half from protein. If we are choosing the most natural meat sources, we will be getting all the essential fats that we need as a natural byproduct of getting our protein requirements.

To top off our calories and stay out of starvation mode, we recommend filling the gap with oils (liquid fats). One tablespoon of oil (whether it's a fish oil supplement, olive oil, coconut oil, etc.) is fourteen grams of fat (120 calories). A tablespoon of oil also isn't that much. We have set up your programs so that we use liquid fats to round out the macronutrients and make sure you get enough of what you need, whether in fat loss or muscle building mode.

If you are concerned that adding fat is a bad thing, we assure you it is not. Every single hormone, cell membrane, and nerve is highly dependent on fats, so they're not something we want to skimp on. Many of the myths surrounding fat intake and its impact on blood lipids and blood cholesterol are unfounded. A report out of the Harvard School of Public Health debunked many of these myths, stating that:

- The total amount of fat in the diet has no real link to weight or disease.
- Sugar and refined carbohydrates are the main contributors to heart disease and diabetes.
- Replacing a carbohydrate-rich diet with one rich in unsaturated fat, predominantly monounsaturated fats, lowers blood pressure, improves lipid levels, and reduces the estimated cardiovascular risk.
- There is insufficient evidence from prospective epidemiologic studies to conclude that dietary saturated fat is associated with an increased risk of coronary heart disease, stroke, or cardiovascular disease. (This study looked at more than 350,000 subjects over twenty-three years.)
- A body of scientific studies shows only a weak relationship between the amount of cholesterol a person consumes and his or her blood cholesterol levels. ★

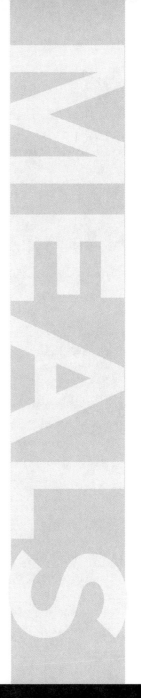

MEALS

Boss to Bikini
90-DAY PROGRAM

OUR NUTRITIONAL PROGRAMS are organized based on the information we've just presented, but they're further broken down by height. Why? Your height determines how much muscle you can carry, and consequently, how much protein or carbs you can effectively use. The fat loss plans will be used for the Ignite and Shred phases, and the maintenance/building plans will be used for the Sculpt phase. You will be required to portion your food so a food scale is necessary. If you think it's too much work, let's look at where you're at from what you were doing previously. Exactly. You still have no idea how to catch a fish! It's time for a change. Every successful fitness model and athlete has a grasp on how much and what type of foods he or she eats. Until you learn, you will not get the results you're after.

Phases of workout and corresponding meal plans

- Ignite: Fat Loss
- Sculpt: Building/Maintenance
- Shred: Fat Loss

In spite of my explanations about how to make food choices that support your goals, I understand that some of you are still overwhelmed. Before you tell me you hate the idea of having to pay attention to macronutrients because it will be too complicated, consider the following:

1. The most successful dieters and athletes have a few "staple" meals that they rotate through consistently and it's easy to figure out the nutritional information of these few meals.

2. YOU ALREADY have staple meals too; most likely, you just haven't figured out their nutritional content.

Find any of the dozens of online nutritional information databases, and figure out the stats behind the healthiest meals that you're already eating. There is no need to re-invent the wheel. Once you figure out your daily requirements, it will be easy to plug your staple meals into the program. This is a great way to start on our programs.

To make things a little easier, I will include some macro nutrient and food guides to help you get the hang of it. I promise after your first week it will be easy breezy!

PROGRAM INSTRUCTIONS

You will have the freedom to choose and prepare the foods you prefer most on this program, as long as you maintain your macro requirements listed in your plan.

In order to be successful, you will need to prepare your food ahead of time. In fitness we call this "meal prep." Preparing your food ahead of time may seem like a hassle at first, but I can assure you it gets easier once you get into a routine. BE PREPARED. If you are not, you will not have success with this program or your goals.

PROGRAM GUIDELINES

1. Eat every two-and-one-half to four hours.

2. Ideal options for veggies:
- Broccoli, spinach, green beans, asparagus, zucchini, Brussel sprouts, spring mix, peppers, cucumbers, celery, onions and all salad greens
- Steam, roast, bake, or grill
- Use oil but make sure you calculate it into your macro allowance. For example: spring mix with one tbsp. of olive oil counts for fourteen grams of fat.
- Avoid starchy veggies like corn, squash, carrots and eggplant.

3. Ideal protein sources
- Lean steak cuts, chicken, turkey breast, egg whites and fish (not tilapia)
- Nuts, seeds, legumes and beans are not ideal sources as discussed earlier.

4. **Carbs**
   - Ideal carb choices—sweet potato, rice, quinoa, non-instant organic oatmeal, organic rice cakes, red potatoes, white potatoes
   - Gluten free pasta is ok on occasion
   - Fruit— Apples, all types of berries, oranges or grapefruit, nectarines, pears, plums, apricots, kiwi – unless others are specified
   - Avoid—breads, pasta, risotto, cereals, wraps, muffins etc.

5. **You should be drinking a gallon of water per day**
   - No more, no less.
   - If you struggle with remembering, get a gallon jug and take it with you all day. It's easier than carrying a bunch of bottles around and it's a constant reminder to drink.

6. **Post Workout (PWO) Meal**
   - Consume this meal within thirty minutes of your training no matter what time of the day you work out.

7. **Free meals**
   - You can have one happy meal per week. (You absolutely need this!)
   - Happy meal is eaten in addition to daily macros.
   - Keep it under 500 calories and keep it semi-clean if possible.

8. **Salt**
   - You should be using sea salt only on your foods. Sodium is a vital electrolyte and you will absolutely need it on this type of training program. Salt will not make you bloated; conversely, avoiding salt will make your body retain water.
   - Do not use table salt. It is a mixture of NaCl and acts differently in the body and usually contains iodine.

9. **Protein powders**

   Not all protein is created equal. Make sure when purchasing protein it is a quality product and not from a mass retailer which is selling low-quality, mass-produced goods. You get what you pay for! I am a big proponent of 1st Phorm products and will include links to my favorite supplements in the appendix.

   Make sure any protein you use is:

   - Gluten free
   - Low carb—under 5g per serving
   - Between 16-24g protein per serving

FOOD RULES – READ AND DIGEST

10. Essential supplements

- Multivitamin
- Omega-3
- Probiotic
- Vitamin D
- Essential amino formula

As I stated earlier, before you start taking supplements, check with your physician, especially if you're already on medication for a specific condition.

Note: See appendix for recommended supplement brands and free shipping link.

General
Shopping Guide > > >

A FEW GUIDELINES for making healthy choices when it comes to food shopping

STRICTLY **AVOID** ANY products with the following ingredients (or using the following wording):

- Glucose, corn syrup, high fructose corn syrup
- Hydrogenated, partially hydrogenated, partially fractionated
- Monosodium glutamate, hydrolyzed vegetable protein, sodium/calcium caseinate, autolyzed yeast extract
- "Natural" or "artificial" flavoring
- Gluten
- Added coloring (e.g.: FD&C No. 1 blue or yellow)
- Aspartame, Saccharin, Sucralose, phenyl alkaline
- Bleached white flour

Food manufacturers try to mislead you with their packaging. The only way to know if something is healthy or not is to read the ingredient list, NOT the front of the package! As a general rule, the fewer ingredients on the label, the better it is for you. Your metabolism will not work efficiently if it is constantly bombarded with processed toxic chemicals from food. EAT FRESH WHOLE FOODS as much as possible. Try to do your shopping on the outside perimeter of the grocery store, avoiding all the aisles of fattening, disease-causing foods. And lastly, if you can't pronounce it, it's probably not good for you. READ THE LABELS!

A note on artificial sweeteners: if you must use a sugar substitute, we recommend Stevia and Xylitol. Just keep in mind that sweet foods will re-ignite our cravings and thus make the program more difficult than it needs to be. My advice: cut sugar cold turkey! Trust me, you will not miss it once it's gone, especially when you see your amazing abs popping out!

Timia Beharry >>

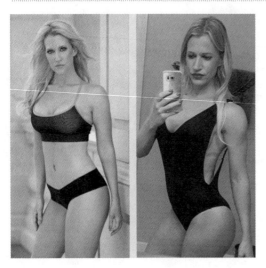

Timia Beharry, age 34

Senior Account Executive

Began working out at age 20, started serious bodybuilding at age 32

Favorite happy meal: Burger and Oreos

"My favorite thing about this type of lifestyle is watching my body respond. What you put into it is what you get out of it. Workouts make me feel physically strong and emotionally happy and satisfied."

Timia's Story: Staying fit was always important to me. While I was in college I was fortunate to have a friend who introduced me to the gym and living a healthy lifestyle. Naturally at that age your metabolism is incredible so with a few adjustments and making the gym a social hour I was always pleased with my body and fitness level. Fast forward eight years and after my second baby, it became more difficult to maintain a fitness regime. Not only does your body change, but priorities do too. I worked so hard to lose the baby weight, but what I had left was still me being skinny fat. So frustrating! I was searching for more. I was on a mission to be fit.

I started my journey by researching online. I trained with one online program; it was a start but not what I desired to achieve. I had several friends that were bikini competitors, however, I actually never considered stepping on stage. What I did know, was that I wanted my body to look like I was [a competitor] and I was determined to achieve it.

I then found Theresa. I instantly clicked with her and trusted she could help me accomplish my goals. I enrolled in her program and became a Bikini Boss Chick. Custom meal plans and workouts, education on nutrition, and guidance on effective supplements. The program not only motivated me but held me accountable. A few months later, Theresa encouraged me to attend a World Beauty Fitness and Fashion (WBFF) show and little did I know my whole world would change from that day on. My passion for fashion was showcased on a glamorous stage with the most fit and beautiful people I have ever seen. The energy was intoxicating. I knew at that moment I found something special, something I wanted to be a part of. I found a deep passion for fitness and nothing would get in my way of achieving my desired goals.

Being a very busy mom of two small children and having a full time career I decided to take on the greatest challenge of my life. I committed to do a WBFF show. Although as an athlete you put in a tremendous amount of sacrifice, so does your family. Hours in the gym, no real social life, and maintaining a household is not easy. The training can be intense and exhausting, some days leaving you with very little energy. As a mom, those days of relaxing and regrouping are no longer an option. I pushed through prepping for several shows and finally became a WBFF pro in October 2015. I achieved a goal I never could have imagined possible!

Now I hope to inspire women who desire to meet a fulfilling goal. Effort will release its reward when you refuse to quit. Bikini Boss Chicks will give you all the tools you need to be successful. What you put into it, you will get out of it. I could not imagine my life without my team or as I better like to think of them, family. I have been educated, made some of my best friends, and shared incredible memories. It was the best decision of my life Instagram @timiatekla

#TheBowlMethod > > >

MANY WOMEN WHO start our program get overwhelmed when first trying to figure out and adapt this style of meal plans to their lives. They tend to over-complicate it and as a result end up getting confused. When you get used to eating this way it is literally the simplest "diet" you will ever follow. That's why it's so easily adapted long-term and becomes part of your lifestyle. "Keep it simple, stupid" is something I often tell clients. You don't need to complicate things to have a great meal. Some of my most favorite dishes have very few ingredients and I'm pretty sure you will agree after you try some of these ideas.

Let's get back to the Basics. At Bikini Boss Fitness, we have coined the term "the bowl method," which is what we use to make different combinations of food (macros) into a delicious meal. We call it the bowl method because you essentially choose one food from each macro groups, toss them in a bowl, top it with your favorite spices, seasonings and/or condiments and voila, you have an amazing meal!

Below I have listed a few of my favorite bowls. These aren't recipes per se because I am not listing specific amounts of food; you will determine the portion size based on your individual meal plans. This is just to get your creative juices flowing and to help you get accustomed to this style of eating. You'll notice I added fat (liquid oil or avocado) to each of these bowls. If you want a meal without a carb or fat macro you could just modify as needed by removing that macro ingredient from the bowl.

FOOD RULES – READ AND DIGEST

BOWL 1
Egg whites
Spring mix
Sweet potato
Olive oil
Vinegar

BOWL 2
Egg whites
Organic oats
Coconut oil
Cinnamon

BOWL 3
Egg whites
Spring mix
Avocado
Garlic
Lemon
Olive oil

BOWL 4
Lean steak
Potato
Bell pepper
Onion
Cilantro
Coconut oil

BOWL 5
Lean steak
White rice
Tomato
Green beans
Basil
Garlic
Olive oil

BOWL 6
Lean steak
Sweet potatoes
Asparagus
MCT oil
Cilantro

BOWL 7
Lean steak
White rice
Onion
Zucchini
Garlic
Coconut amino
Ginger
Green onion

BOWL 8
Ground turkey or beef
Taco seasoning
White rice
Salsa
Cilantro
Avocado

BOWL 9
Ground turkey
White rice
Tomato sauce
Basil
Garlic
Olive oil

BOWL 10
Ground turkey meatballs (cut up)
Sweet potato
Cauliflower

BOSS TO BIKINI

Thyme
Garlic
Olive oil

BOWL 11
Grilled/ baked chicken
Spring mix
Sweet potatoes
Olive oil
Vinegar

BOWL 12
Grilled/ baked chicken
Zucchini
Onions and tomatoes
White potato
Basil
Olive oil

BOWL 13
Grilled/ baked chicken
Spinach
Onions
Asparagus
Olive oil
Vinegar

BOWL 14
Wild Salmon
White rice
Broccoli
Onion
Ginger
Garlic
Coconut oil
Coconut amino

BOWL 15
Baked White fish
White potatoes
Old bay
Parsley and/or onions
Peppers
Garlic
Olive

Lastly, one of the most difficult things for people to adapt to with this type of program is what to eat for breakfast. Here is a rule—most of the typical breakfast foods are terrible for you. Period. We want to avoid processed foods like cereals, instant oats and waffles, etc. To be successful with this program and lifestyle, get rid of the entire "breakfast" notion to begin with. We eat MEALS several times a day. No snacks, no lunch, no breakfast. For example, I personally like egg whites for my first meal (protein) and I typically eat them on a salad (veggie) with oil and vinegar (fat). You can see how I got all of my macros in for that meal. If you had a carb you could add sweet potatoes etc. I also sometimes make eggs over veggies or mix up a smoothie with 1st Phorm level 1 (protein), avocado (fat), spinach (veggies) and berries (carbs). So as long as you're getting your macros for that meal you can get creative.

147

CHAPTER 11

Using Every Tool in Our Toolbox

IF YOU'VE BEEN reading all the chapters carefully, you have learned that there is a difference between eating and training for health and eating and training for aesthetics. Not understanding this difference is the reason many of you will fail. If you're not familiar with the word aesthetic, let me clarify. Aesthetic, in fitness, refers to the way things look, rather than how they function. When it comes to being healthy and feeling good, any type of movement and a diet of whole foods will suffice. However, when it comes to optimizing hormones, building muscle, and burning fat, we have to get a lot more precise use out of every tool we have in our tool box because, let's face it, women are not designed to carry as much lean muscle as we are attempting to have. We are genetically programmed to hold more fat than men, evolutionarily speaking, so we can ensure the best chance of survival for our offspring during gestation and nursing. Therefore, when we want to make these types of changes we need to go beyond simply "being healthy." That's not to say health isn't one of our primary goals because it is. But what most people deem "healthy" will not get you the body you're seeking. What we are going to do takes much more effort—both in terms of physical activity and diet—than what you have done in the past. But you already know this.

We have to make sure your body has what it needs—when it needs it—to be able to do all of the things we're trying to accomplish. Obviously, following your meal plan is an integral part of this program, but as we have learned from earlier chapters, we cannot always count on the quality of food or the ability of our body to optimally absorb what we are eating. As such, supplementation plays a significant role in the success of our programs and post-workout supplementation is paramount to maximize the results from your workout. I have already discussed the supplements required for overall metabolic health, but now I'm going to explain in detail the importance of proper post-workout nutrition.

THE REAL DEAL ON POST-WORKOUT SUPPLEMENTATION

I'm often asked about the best kind of post-workout supplementation, and while the truth is "the best" will be different for each of you depending on your goals, there are some universal rules which apply to everyone. When I look at what's best for one's body and metabolism, I think about how our bodies are designed to eat and move from a physiological standpoint. I find when you do things that follow the natural processes of the body, you get optimal results, not just in fitness and fat loss but in overall health as well.

First, let's discuss our post-workout physiology because understanding this gives us the advantage when it comes to nutrient timing.

From an evolutionary perspective, the human body was not designed to undergo long bouts of intense exercise or heavy lifting but instead was made for rather short, extremely high intensity physical demands such as sprinting from or fighting off the proverbial saber-toothed tiger. These extreme "workouts" were followed by long rest periods to recover. Our genes—and therefore metabolic pathways—evolved to be able to provide our bodies with the necessary hormones and subsequent energy to survive these extreme physical demands. Enter the "fight or flight" response—our bodies' natural sympathetic nervous system response to a stressor. As discussed earlier, this involuntary response sets off a cascade of events which starts with your adrenal glands and ends with your pancreas signaling to flood the body with blood sugar and shunt blood to the extremities to be able to fight or run away.

So what does this mean to YOU? When you do intense exercise such as sprinting or lifting heavy weights, your body reacts as if it's in a state of "fight or flight." Your brain reacts appropriately by signaling your body to send all of your blood to your extremities to be able to tackle the physical demand which ultimately shuts down your digestion and floods the body with sugars (i.e., glucose). This process is in place to make sure you've got enough energy for fight (exercise) or flight (run away) because the body does not know the difference between a 45-minute cardio session and a 45-minute hunt for a tiger. While you definitely want to eat within the 30- to

45-minute (anabolic, aka "building stuff") window to replenish glycogen and protein stores, you also want to make sure you are feeding your body with the CORRECT type of nutrients and protein which can be absorbed easily since digestion is impaired. So, understanding this reaction helps us to discern this universal rule:

SO WHAT SHOULD YOU EAT?

The goal of your post-workout supplementation is the following:

1: You actually want to elicit an insulin spike. We accomplish this by consuming a high glycemic carbohydrate. It's the ONLY time when a high glycemic carb is beneficial because the insulin basically acts like a school bus that shuttles the protein into the cells. Without it, there is no way for protein to get in. Although foods such as rice and potatoes are carbohydrates and can eventually be broken down into glucose, it's not ideal to eat them post-workout because – remember – our digestion is impaired. Those carbohydrates fall under the category of di/tri- saccharides, meaning in order to be utilized for energy, they still need to be broken down by a process called dehydration synthesis, or as we know it, digestion. You want to eat a carbohydrate that is already broken down so that you will get an effective and immediate insulin spike. This type of carbohydrate is called a mono-saccharide and is ideal in a post-workout setting only. There are different types of mono-saccharide supplements available so just make sure you purchase one from a reputable company as discussed in chapter 8. (I will include a link to all of my personal favorite supplements in appendix B.)

2: Since digestion is slowed, it doesn't make sense to eat a whole foods protein source such as animal meat or fish, etc. We want to make sure we give our bodies the best chance for absorption by taking a hydrolyzed protein (partially broken down) which will allow us to bypass the digestive process and be ready for assimilation. If you're eating whole foods or non- hydrolyzed protein you're not going to get the most benefit from your workouts because your body will not be able to digest the protein efficiently enough to acquire the nutrients necessary for optimal results.

Taken TOGETHER, these two steps will allow your body to take in nutrients, increase glycogen and intra-cellular protein, and rapidly repair your muscles, thus helping to increase your metabolism and ultimately speeding up fat loss.

With regard to post-workout nutrition macros, "the best" varies according to your current conditioning level, training program, and desired outcome. I would suggest centering your carbs mainly around your workouts for the day regardless of the phase. This would mean eating a good portion of your carbs pre and post workout.

We have designed your meal plans with this in mind so it's best to stick with the macros and order of meals we provided. ★

Margarita McKibben >>

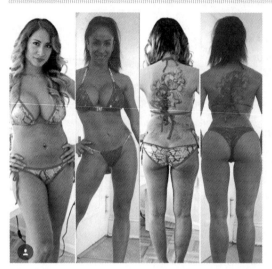

Margarita McKibben, age 35

Fitness Model & Entertainer; Fitness, Fashion

First workout: Dance at age 3/ Gym at age 6

Favorite happy meal: Pizza because I don't consider a burger a 'cheat' meal (lol)

My favorite thing about this type of lifestyle is the constant evolution of goals and transformation inside and out. Workouts make me feel empowered and have self-realization."

Margarita's Story: I became a client of Bikini Boss Fitness a few years ago around the time Theresa walked the runway during my athletic fashion show during New York Fashion Week. She was a spokesmodel for my online fashion boutique at that time and we quickly hit it off. I took a leap and decided to compete at a WBFF show and started training to become one of her Regional Assistant Coaches. I loved that woman from the get-go and would do just about anything to support her mission; not surprisingly, this is the same devotion you will find among Bikini Boss Fitness clients and staff members. This by far is the sign that Theresa and BBF is one of those rare gems you don't often find today.

Before Bikini Boss Fitness, I struggled with understanding my hormones and damaged metabolism due to fad diets and over-training that I did in the past, which I didn't realize was holding me back. I was already athletic and dedicated to fitness but I did not understand the science of food and supplements in combination with workouts. She's created comprehensive programs that are flexible to my ever-changing busy schedule. She also fosters clients to become more educated and empowered within their own transformation.

Among the things I have learned is the importance of a post-workout regimen; somehow I had missed that memo in the past, along with the importance of avoiding further damage to my thyroid and metabolism. I really didn't know much about these two things, but they have helped me tremendously to reach my goals.

I also learned so much about food and its effects on my body, since BBF's plans are not cookie cutter but allow you to pick and choose your meals based on macros while helping you become more knowledgeable about macro nutrients. As a modern woman, understanding your hormones in relation to food and your workouts makes all the difference in the world.

If you're struggling and considering starting this program, I would say that you are given one life and the good one is the one that you make for yourself. One of the greatest investments you can make is in your health. If you're looking for a comprehensive program that also complements your ever-changing busy life, then this is the program for you. You'll learn so much about nutrition and fitness and also the power within yourself. Transformation of any kind is never easy. The constant support, compassion, and camaraderie of Bikini Boss Fitness is invaluable. There's no time like the present to invest in yourself because you are so worth it! MargaritaMcKibben.com

CHAPTER 12

Frequently Asked Questions

TRAINING QUESTIONS:

Q Does it matter what time of the day you work out?

A No. Whatever works best for you and your schedule! As long as you get it in.

Q Is there any cardio during Phase 1 of the 90-Day program?

A This workout is a conditioning-style workout; this means you will be getting an intense cardiovascular workout with the exercises given.

NOTE: Sunday is active recovery day for everyone—meaning you are free to take a forty-five-minute walk, leisurely bike ride or swim, play basketball, soccer, etc. As we explained previously, walking is encouraged.

Q If you're doing an early morning workout (as soon as you wake up), do you work out on an empty stomach or not? If not (which I'm sure is the case), what can you eat and do you have to wait a certain period of time before working out?

A Eat within thirty minutes of waking up! You need to plan your day and schedule around your meals. If you need more time, wake up earlier.

P.S. If it were easy – everyone would be doing it. No excuses :)

Q Are there any modifications for lunge jumps or any jump exercises? My knees have a tendency to bother me and I don't want to injure myself. The lunge jumps seem to bother me more.

A Yes, just do a squat or lunge or whatever the movement is without jumping.

Q Are you getting the most from your workouts?

A You've heard me discuss making sure you are keeping your intensity up during your workouts. This is accomplished by making sure you're using an appropriate weight and also by brief rest periods.

Q How do you know what an appropriate weight is?

A The easiest way to know what weight is best is by this simple rule:

You should be using a weight heavy enough that you can barely get through your last few reps. In fact, I often have to take a brief rest in between the reps to be able to finish. And that's okay! (By brief I'm talking about less than five seconds.) Having to take a forced rest means the weight is heavy and challenging enough to get results—which is the goal of the workout. If you're flying through the reps without having to stop, you need to increase your weight. Another way to maximize your workouts is by taking brief rest periods and using a higher tempo of speed for your reps. In all your workouts, I have specified the appropriate rest time to get you the most benefit with adequate recovery so you'll be able to do your next set. Stick with the guidelines I gave you and you'll be good. If it says thirty seconds rest between sets, don't rest for five minutes. If you're new to lifting and you need longer rest at first, that's okay but make it your goal to decrease your rest time as you go on.

Lastly, even though you're doing the same workout plan for four weeks you should ALWAYS be progressing:

- Increase your weight
- Add progressions
- Decrease rest, if you've been taking longer than the recommended time.

You shouldn't be doing the exact same thing over and over. I recommend printing out your workouts and bringing them with you to the gym on a clipboard so you can keep track of the weight you're lifting each week. It's a great way to gauge your progress.

MEAL PLAN/FOOD FAQ:

Q I see fish under approved protein but not tilapia. Is there a reason why?

A YES! Tilapia is now exclusively a farm-raised fish. This variety no longer exists in the wild. Because of this, the quality and health of the fish suffer dramatically due to being caged with hundreds—sometimes thousands—of other fish. They get sick and transfer diseases so they have to be fed antibiotics (which accumulate in tissues that you eat). They can't move as well, making them unhealthy; they easily acquire parasites because of their poor health which is why it's not uncommon to find worms in them; and their nutritional value becomes more detrimental than beneficial. If you can find a LOCAL ORGANICALLY raised farmed tilapia that is acceptable, but they're also very rare and expensive. Try to stick with the other choices I've listed on your grocery list.

Q Liquid fats, must I have them? Can I use them?

A Yes, you absolutely need to make sure you are consuming all your fats. You should be eating only super lean meats so we measure fats separately to keep it precise. I always use one of my servings of fat per day as fish oil—so take one tablespoon of fish oil per day. The others you should try to choose from your food guide.

Q Should I weigh my carbs?

A The only carb we weigh on a scale is potatoes.

For all other carbs except potatoes we go by the package label.

For example: if the serving size is one cup = fifty grams of carbs, half a cup would be twenty-five grams and so on. Always go by whatever the label says based on the serving size.

For potatoes, if you're using a scale, one ounce of potato = six grams carbs

Q Can we change the order of when we eat the carbs with our meal? For example, I have lunch (which is my meal two) at my office around noon. I have more time to eat then. I will eat my meal three around three or four o'clock (I don't get a break then, so I have to eat quickly). It would be easier for me to have the carbs with meal two instead of meal three. Can we change when we eat them, as long as the total carbs for the day stay the same?

A Yes, as long as you keep the post-workout meal (shake + ignition) in place you can move around meals if absolutely necessary. We organize the meals to get you the maximum benefit from your plan so I would suggest following as closely as possible

Q Can we have avocados?

A You can eat them but you have to count them towards your fat total.

Q If we want to drink coffee and add almond milk, how would we calculate that into our macros?

A If you use almond milk it's negligible. If you use coconut I would count that toward fat. As a general rule, black coffee is ideal, but if you must add something, use unsweetened almond and coconut milk. Processed soy and dairy creamers are a no-no. Sugar-free syrups fall under Red light category, too.

Q When we use fish oil, can we take

the pills if that's easier instead of cutting them all open and pouring them on our food?

A Yes but in order to know how many to take, you need to cut them open and measure first.

For example, four of the Full Mega caps = one tbsp. = fourteen grams

Q What do we eat or drink to replace the post-workout meal on rest days?

A You can replace with whole foods on rest days. You should be getting all of your macros in every day so you still need to eat the two meal macros even on rest days

Q Can we put lemons in our gallon of water?

A Absolutely!

Q Thoughts on lamb and veal for protein?

A Any protein less than three percent fat is ideal. If you decide to choose a fattier cut you need to take into account the fat in your fat total for the day.

Q I have terrible sweet cravings in the afternoon. What do you suggest I do?

A It will pass; your body is releasing toxins. Drink an extra protein shake if you need to, it will help; especially the 1st Phorm brand because it tastes like a treat. Secondly, make sure you are taking all of your supplements. Cravings are usually indicative of an underlying adrenal issue, especially in the afternoon.

Q Will Greek yogurt ever be allowed as a protein?

A No dairy is a protein.

Q Since I know sparkling water is approved how often can you drink it?

A As often as you wish

Q What are some good snacks to have handy when your planned two-hour round trip appointment turns into five hours? How do we prepare for the unexpected?

A We don't eat snacks because we eat five to six meals a day. Get the idea of snacks out of your head. To be successful you need to think ahead about how you can get in your meals on the day and plan accordingly. For an unexpected occasion, a protein shake would work well.

Q I have stuck to my plan, to the T, and

am now at a banquet for work. I have my last meal packed in the car. This is a sit down dinner. I don't know how I'm going to manage to sneak out of here and eat MY food in my car and not touch what they feed us tonight!

A Well you have two options. You can try to eat the healthiest options available or you can bring in your food. There is usually always a way to survive a dinner out without being totally destructive. Pass on the bread and butter and ask for sauces on the side, etc.

Q If we know we won't be eating for more than four hours, when is the best time to take the anabolic bridge supplement you recommend? At the three-hour mark? I work in a diner and I eat my breakfast between 5:30 and 6:30 and work until noon and I don't have time to sit and eat during that time.

A Yes, that works. Any time after the three-hour window will help you avoid muscle wasting

Q I reviewed the list of approved foods and saw that vinegar is not an approved condiment. Is it okay to use?

A Yes, vinegar is totally fine.

Q Thoughts on lentils for protein?

A Refer to chapter 10 but lentils are not ideal. It says on your grocery list to avoid beans and legumes. The ratio of protein/carbs is very high so it's not just protein. In addition, they can become inflammatory.

Q I made turkey burgers last night with 99% fat free ground turkey, but they came out kind of dry since there isn't any fat to moisten it up. Are there any tricks you guys have to keep the turkey from getting dry? (I grilled them on the George Forman grill.)

A You can use "ground turkey" not just the breast but you have to account for the fat in your fat for that meal. Also if you want you can add oil into meat before you cook—I use extra virgin olive oil. Again just count into your fat total for that meal.

Q For chicken, if I use leg quarters, would I have to calculate the fat in it for my macros as well, and what about whole eggs?

A Yes and yes. Count fat for both, for dark meat and whole egg. Egg whites are all protein so you don't have to calculate fat.

Q Is it normal to feel bloated? Although I can see I'm a little tighter and even feel a little tighter, I have been feeling a little bloated the last few days and I don't think I have really changed anything.

A Two considerations:

1. Make sure you are drinking all of your water.
2. Make sure you're salting your food.

When you work out hard and increase water intake it is crucial you get salt which is an electrolyte. You don't want to use table salt which is sodium chloride. You want to use pure sea salt (sodium).

Q Regarding the happy meal, this is ON TOP of our regular meal plan for the day, correct? So it is basically 500 calories more to my daily plan, right?

A Yes! In addition to your normal meals—one day per week.

Q I try not to eat protein bars, but occasionally it is my only option for a meal. I always try to eat an actual meal if I can. However, is there a particular protein bar you recommend above others if I must eat one sometimes?

A To be totally honest they are all terrible. My best advice would be to drink a protein shake and mix oatmeal in it for carbs (if you have them in that meal) and take fish oil for fat or maybe double up one of your meals later after you can eat again. (Remember the meal frequency myth: It is the total number of macros which matters most.)

SUPPLEMENT QUESTIONS

Q I ordered the supplements you recommended but I had just bought another large thing of protein right before. Is it okay if I order the Phormula 1 after I use the one I have?

A Yes, Absolutely! Use what you have and you can order Phormula 1 after.

Q I started taking Thyro-Drive and feel very hungry. Is this normal?

A 1) YES! It's normal to feel hungrier and warm. That's a good thing; it means your metabolism is working!!

2) Thyro-Drive is designed to give your thyroid all the nutrients it needs to function optimally which is why we take it in addition to our programs—to give us an extra metabolic boost! Make sure you are cycling five days with two days off. Repeat!

3) Is it safe to take it if I have a thyroid condition? Yes, you can take it if you have hypothyroidism. The only contraindication would be an autoimmune condition like *Hashimoto's* disease.

Q What makes a good protein powder?

A I'm sure most of you have tried a protein powder and gotten really bloated and gassy after. There is a very specific reason for that. Ninety-nine percent of the supplement brands that make protein use high temperature heat processing because it is cheaper and faster to produce which means they can make more product and more sales for the company. The problem is that high temperature heat processing denatures the protein beyond the point of recognition so your body has a very difficult time digesting and absorbing it. This is why when you drink it, the bacteria in your intestines attack all the undigested protein passing through your gut and produce a ton of gas as a by-product, leaving you bloated as hell and gassy. The worst part—lacking results. If you ever wonder why old school body builders (and some current) eat raw eggs all the time this is the reason. The more natural the state of the protein (meaning not denatured) the better your body can absorb it. This is one of the many reasons I use 1st Phorm because the company uses cool-temperature processed proteins. Many people, including yours truly, are able to actually tolerate it because they do not get that same horrible reaction they get from others. Also, you'll notice a night-and-day difference using quality protein because your body is able to absorb it. The results are ridiculous!

Lastly, I touched on this previously but with ANY supplements—you want to make sure they are produced in an FDA-approved lab. There is no such thing as an FDA-approved supplement. The FDA doesn't approve supplements. The highest quality and best supplement brands are those with FDA-inspected lab sticker on the label because it means they have been tested to make sure processing and manufacturing is what they say it is.

Q What are some important supplements for brain function?

A Believe it or not three of the most important nutrients for brain function are a multivitamin, probiotic, and omega-3 (full mega). Here's why:

1) The myelin sheath is what surrounds the nerve cells and transmits nerve impulses from the brain (afferent) and to the brain (efferent) and a deficiency of omega-3 causes massive interruptions and inhibits the speed and efficiency of impulses

2) Omega-3 constitutes the majority of cell membrane of ALL cells in our body. This goes for skin, hair, nails, muscles, nerve, and brain. You get the gist. Deficiency of omega-3 causes major issues with cell-wall permeability, affecting the ability of nutrients to get into the cell and ultimately impairing the cell from proper metabolism and function. This is why I stress the importance of omega-3 for fat loss and fitness results, but the truth is it's essential for Health.

3) The vast majority of brain tissue (white matter) is made of fat—specifically DHA which is a component of omega-3.

4) Inflammation is one of the main causes of poor brain function—this is caused primarily by poor diet, one void of

omega-3 and filled with processed foods rich in omega-6. Omega-3 reduces systemic inflammation and subsequently improves brain function.

5) Then there is the gut–brain connection. What we currently know is a properly functioning gut is paramount to proper brain function. They call the gut the "second brain" for a reason. The typical American diet breeds an unhealthy and unbalanced gut leading to inflammation, gut permeability and neurological disorders such as ADD, depression, and auto-immune disorders. An innate diet (like our program) with probiotics can help restore order to the gut and reduce inflammation.

6) Multivitamins act as co-factors and co-enzymes for all metabolic processes in the body. Basically, they are catalysts for cellular metabolism. This includes neurotransmitter function, neural function, and some of the major components of brain function.

This is why most of my clients (the ones who listen and take the supplements I recommend) report they have improved mental clarity and focus as two of the major side effects of this program. For you moms out there—this is the reason you should also give your kids these supplements as well. ★

APPENDICES

GROCERY LIST

This is a list of approved foods for your program. You are free to choose foods you prefer from this list for your meal plan. The foods on the list are categorized by macronutrient to help you follow the program's guidelines.

Beverages

- Unsweetened almond milk
- Unsweetened coconut milk
- Purified water
- Sparkling water
- Coffee (not pre-made)
- Tea—unsweetened
- Avoid: artificially sweetened drinks, sweetened drinks, artificial coloring or flavors

Protein

- Lean red meat (three percent fat or less)
- Hormone-free chicken breast
- Ground turkey
- Fish: salmon, grouper, flounder, sea bass, cod, Arctic char, fluke
- Egg whites (organic, cage-free)
- Canned tuna, preservative free (use sparingly)
- Avoid: fatty cuts, farm-raised fish, shell fish, non-organic free range meat

Carbohydrates

- Potatoes: red, white, sweet
- Organic non-instant oatmeal
- Organic rice, white or brown (plain)
- Quinoa
- Avoid: beans and processed carbs such as crackers, etc.

Carbs cont'd: Fruit

- Blueberries
- Strawberries
- Blackberries
- Raspberries
- Oranges
- Grapefruit

195

- Apples
- Avoid: high glycemic choices including bananas, pineapples, mango, grapes, and melon (post-workout is the only exception)

Vegetables

- Green beans
- Asparagus
- Zucchini
- Brussels sprouts
- Spinach
- Broccoli
- Cauliflower
- Escarole
- Broccoli rabe
- Cucumber
- Peppers
- Celery
- Onion
- Tomato
- Mushrooms
- All green leafy lettuce
- Avoid: carrots, peas, squash, corn, artichokes

Fats

- Olive oil
- Coconut oil
- MCT oil
- Fish oil (see supplement info sheet)
- Avocado

Condiments/spices extras (Use sparingly)

- Organic yellow mustard
- Organic ketchup (low sugar)
- Gluten free organic marinades
- Tabasco/ hot sauce
- Sea salt
- Pepper
- Garlic
- All spices approved

Extras

- Tin foil
- Zip lock bags
- Meal-size Tupperware
- Protein shakers
- Canola spray
- Plastic to-go forks

There are no FDA approved supplements. The safest and most effective supplements you can take are made at an FDA approved lab. As with any diet or exercise program, always consult your physisican before you start taking any supplements, especially if you are being treated for any serious medical conditions.

Here are my recommended Supplements:

1st Phorm Products

- **Phormula 1**—Ideal as pre/post workout protein because of its rapid assimilation and high BCAA content. (counts as protein)
- **Full Mega Omega-3 supplement**—helps fight inflammation and regulate hormones and metabolism
- **Adrenal Restore** – helps prevent and repair adrenal fatigue issues and optimizes fat loss and energy.

- **Anabolic bridge**—excellent supplement to help prevent muscle wasting at night and ideal for clients who have to go long periods between meals due to work/school etc.
- **Thyro-Drive**—gives the body essential nutrients to balance thyroid for optimal metabolic effects. Is not a fat burner or stimulant.
- **M-factor goddess**—multivitamin, super foods and antioxidants and essential amino acids. Everything your body needs to be able to functions at its highest metabolic peak
- **Ignition**—Recovery supplement to be used post-workout with Phormula 1 protein (counts as carb)

Free Shipping Link for all Boss to Bikini readers:

WWW.BIKINIBOSSSUPPLEMENTS.COM

1. Ratey, John J., and Richard Manning. *Go Wild: Free Your Body and Mind from the Afflictions of Civilization.* New York: Little, Brown and Company. 2014.

2. Magnusson, S. Peter, and Erik B. Simonsen, Peter Aagaard, and Michael Kjaer. "Biomechanical responses to repeated stretches in human hamstring muscle in vivo." *The American Journal of Sports Medicine.* 24: 622-628. September-October 1996.

3. Magnusson, S.P., and P. Aagaard, B. Larsson and M. Kjaer. "Passive energy absorption by human muscle-tendon unit is unaffected by increase in intramuscular temperature." *Journal of Applied Physiology.* 88: 1215-1220. April 2000.

4. Magnusson S.P., and E.B. Simonsen, P. Aagaard, H. Sorensen, and M. Kjaer. "A mechanism for altered flexibility in human skeletal muscle." *The Journal of Physiology.* 497: 291-298. Nov. 15, 1996.

5. O'Keefe, James H., and Robert Vogel, Carl J. Lavie, and Loren Cordain. "Achieving Hunter-gatherer Fitness in the 21st Century: Back to the Future." *The American Journal of Medicine.* 123(12): 1082-86. December 2010.

6. Mohler, Betty J., and William B. Thompson, Sarah H. Creem-Regehr, Herbert L. Pick, Jr., and William H. Warren, Jr. "Visual flow influences gait transition speed and preferred walking speed." *Experimental Brain Research* 181(2): 221–228. March 2007.

7. Kraemer, William J., and Jeff S. Volek, Kristine L. Clark, Scott E. Gordon, Susan M. Puhl, L. Perry Koziris, Jeffrey M. McBride, N. Travis Triplett-McBride, Margot Putukian, Robert U. Newton, Keijo Hakkinen,

Jill A. Bush, and Wayne J. Sebastianelli. "Influence of exercise training on physiological and performance changes with weight loss in men." *Medicine & Science in Sports & Exercise.* 31(9): 1320-1329. September 1999.

8. Hagan, R. Donald, and S. Jill Upton, Les Wong, and James Whittam. "The effects of aerobic conditioning and/or caloric restriction in overweight men and women." *Medicine & Science in Sports & Exercise.* 18(1): 87-94. February 1996.

9. Chaitow Leon, Christopher Gilbert, and Dinah Bradley. *Recognizing and Treating Breathing Disorders: A Multidisciplinary Approach, Second Edition.* Edinburgh: Churchill Livingstone Elsevier. 2013.

10. Body Recomposition. *What's my genetic muscular potential?* 2009. http://www.bodyrecomposition.com/muscle-gain/whats-my-genetic-muscular-potential.html/

11. Zoë Harcombe: Diet, obesity, nutrition & big business: so much, so wrong. "1lb does not equal 3500 calories" 2011. http://www.zoeharcombe.com/standalone/1lb-does-not-equal-3500-calories/

12. Keys, Ancel, Josef Brožek, Austin Henschel, Olaf Mickelsen, and Henry Longstreet Taylor. *The Biology of Human Starvation. Volume I and Volume II.* Minneapolis. The University of Minnesota Press. 1950.

13. Wikipedia. *Basal Metabolic Rate.* Last modified December 2015. http://en.wikipedia.org/wiki/Basal_metabolic_rate

14. World Health Organization. WHO definition of Health. Last modified August 24, 2010. http://www.who.int/about/definition/en/print.html

15. Indiana University. *Obesity, Type 2 Diabetes, and Fructose.* http://www.indiana.edu/~oso/Fructose/Fructose.html

16. Nikpartow, Nick, and Adrienne D. Danyliw, Susan J. Whiting, Hyum Lim, and Hassanali Vatanparast. "Fruit drink consumption is associated with overweight and obesity in Canadian women." *The Canadian Journal of Public Health.* 103(3): 178-82. May-June, 2012.

17. Huffington Post. *Toxic Sugar: Should We Regulate It Like Alcohol?* Last modified February 3, 2012. http://www.huffingtonpost.com/2012/02/02/sugar-toxic-regulation_n_1248397.html

18. YouTube. *Sugar: The Bitter Truth.* July 30, 2009. http://www.youtube.com/watch?v=dBnniua6-oM

19. Wikipedia. *Trans fat*. Last modified January 9, 2016. http://en.wikipedia.org/wiki/Trans_fats

20. Lanou, Amy Joy. "Should dairy be recommended as part of a healthy vegetarian diet? Counterpoint[1,2,3]." *The American Journal of Clinical Nutrition*. 89(5): 1638S-1642S. May 2009.

21. Bertron P., N.D. Barnard, and M. Mills. "Racial bias in federal nutrition policy, Part I: The public health implications of variations in lactase persistence. *Journal of the National Medical Association*. 91(3): 151-57. March 1999.

22. ABC News. *Sixty Percent of Adults Can't Digest Milk*. 2013. http://abcnews.go.com/Health/WellnessNews/story?id=8450036

23. Burke, Louise M. "Caffeine and sports performance." *Applied Physiology, Nutrition, and Metabolism*. 33(6): 1319-1334. December 6, 2008. http://www.nrcresearchpress.com/doi/abs/10.1139/h08-130#citart1

24. Devasagayam T.P.A., J.P. Kamat, Hari Mohan, and P.C. Kesavan. "Caffeine as an antioxidant: inhibition of lipid peroxidation induced by reactive oxygen species." *Biochimica et Biophysica Acta (BBA)—Biomembranes*. 1282(13): 63–70. June 1996. http://www.sciencedirect.com/science/article/pii/0005273696000405

25. Smith, Andrew, David Sutherland, and Gary Christopher. "Effects of repeated doses of caffeine on mood and performance of alert and fatigued volunteers." *Journal of Psychopharmacology*. 19(6): 620-626. November 2005. http://jop.sagepub.com/content/19/6/620.short

26. Somani, S.M., and P. Gupta. "Caffeine: a new look at an age-old drug." *International Journal of Clinical Pharmacology, Therapy, and Toxicology*. 26(11): 521-533. 1988. http://ukpmc.ac.uk/abstract/MED/3072303reload=0;jsessionid=FBmjHrMU6mGmsP21aaa6.24

27. Wolf, Robb. *The Paleo Solution: The Original Human Diet*. Las Vegas: Victory Belt Publishing. 2010.

28. WebMD. "Protein: Are You Getting Enough?" Last modified September 5, 2014. http://www.webmd.com/food-recipes/protein

29. Phillips, Stuart M., and Luc J.C. "Dietary protein for athletes: From requirements to optimum adaptation." *Journal of Sports Sciences*. 29(Supplement 1): S29-S38. 2011. http://www.tandfonline.com/doi/full/10.1080/02640414.2011.619204

30. Body Recomposition. "Meal Frequency and Energy Balance." 2015. http://www.bodyrecomposition.com/research-review/meal-frequency-and-energy-balance-research-review.html

31. Harvard School of Public Health. "Fats and Cholesterol." http://www.hsph.harvard.edu/nutritionsource/what-should-you-eat/fats-and-cholesterol/

BOSS TO BIKINI

For more on Theresa and the 90 Day program, visit her website
bikinibossfitness.com
where you'll find great information on diet, exercise,
and staying motivated.

Connect with me on social!

Snapchat: BikiniBoss
Facebook: Theresa DePasquale
Instagram: @BikiniBossTheresa
Twitter: @BikiniBoss